A Colour Atlas of

The Newborn

R.D.G. Milner
MA, MD, PhD, ScD, FRCP

Professor and Head, Department of Paediatrics,
University of Sheffield

S.M. Herber
MB, BCh, MRCP

Clinical Research Fellow, Department of Paediatrics,
University of Sheffield

Wolfe Medical Publications Ltd

Copyright © R.D.G. Milner & S.M. Herber, 1984
Published by Wolfe Medical Publications Ltd, 1984
Printed by Royal Smeets Offset b.v., Weert, Netherlands
ISBN 0 7234 0742 8

This book is one of the titles in the series of
Wolfe Medical Atlases, a series which brings
together probably the world's largest systematic
published collection of diagnostic
photographs.
For a full list of Atlases in the series, plus
forthcoming titles and details of our surgical,
dental and veterinary Atlases, please write to
Wolfe Medical Publications Ltd, Wolfe House,
3 Conway Street, London W1P 6HE.

General Editor, Wolfe Medical Atlases:
G. Barry Carruthers, MD(Lond)

Contents

Acknowledgements

We wish to thank Mrs J. Gellipter and Dr J. Tsanakas for editorial assistance and the Department of Medical Illustration at the Northern General Hospital and Royal Hallamshire Hospital, Sheffield for their help with the photography. We are most grateful and indebted to Sue Ibbotson for her patient typing of the text.

The Atlas would not have been possible without the generous co-operation of the following colleagues who provided the slides to illustrate it:

J. A. Black

C. E. Blank

S. S. Bleehen

A. W. Boon

J. A. S. Dickson

J. L. Emery

R. R. Gordon

W. T. Houlsby

R. S. Illingworth

R. K. Levick

J. S. Lilleyman

E. A. MacKinnon

M. J. Patrick

R. G. Pearse

B. L. Priestley

R. A. Primhak

G. Russell

S. A. W. Salfield

J. W. Scopes

L. Spitz

D. Stoker

L. S. Taitz

D. Tomovic

G. Whincup

M. F. Whitfield

R. B. Zachary

Preface

This Atlas is a compilation of clinical and radiological illustrations put together for the benefit of all who care for the newborn infant, doctor and nurse alike. Neonatology is characterized by a small number of common signs such as cyanosis, fits and jaundice and a large number of unusual or rare signs. The common signs have individually a low diagnostic precision whereas the rarer signs may often be pathognomonic. Clinical acumen depends partly on logical deduction but also on lateral association and it is clear that the student of neonatology needs to see as many clinical conditions as possible to have the spectrum of information that will equip him to deduce and associate effectively. It is for this purpose that the Atlas has been prepared.

In bringing the slides together we found that our colleagues with collections had, as philatelists do, a large amount of material in common and the occasional gem of their own. The value of the book rests heavily on their generosity in making the material available to us and thereby to the reader who has immediately a vast range of neonatal conditions that would be encountered in clinical practice only after many years of experience.

We are conscious that there is no end to such a collection and the decision to stop compiling and to assemble the book was based on our desire to produce a relatively inexpensive Atlas that would be a useful learning aid. It has been our intention that the Atlas and a textbook of neonatology should be used in a complementary fashion. As every student knows, when he is too tired to read he can still look at the pictures.

1 The whole baby

The first chapter has been called "The whole baby" to illustrate aspects of neonatology that are of general significance. The importance of looking at each infant to assess the appropriateness of growth for gestational age cannot be over emphasized. Expertise in this initial appraisal of a baby will help greatly in the analysis of what may ail the infant. Neonatology is characterized by a relatively small number of common physical signs which may be the result of a wide variety of pathologies. Examples such as hypotonia and oedema are illustrated in this chapter and the illustrations are loosely linked by association since the skill of clinical diagnosis is a fine balance between logical analysis and lateral thinking.

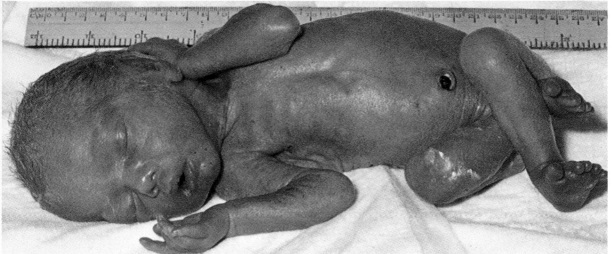

1 A pre-term infant. Gestational age is divided into pre-term (less than 259 days or 37 weeks from the first day of the last menstrual period), term (259 to 286 days inclusive) and post-term (287 or more days or 41 or more weeks). This slide shows a pre-term infant of 32 weeks gestation who is of appropriate weight. Note the smooth skin, the generalized pink colour due to lack of subcutaneous fat and the semi-flexed posture of the limbs. Other important physical characteristics of a pre-term infant include the cartilage in the external auricle, the breast bud, the external genitalia and the degree of creasing of the sole of the feet, and critical assessment of these helps in the estimation of gestational age.

2

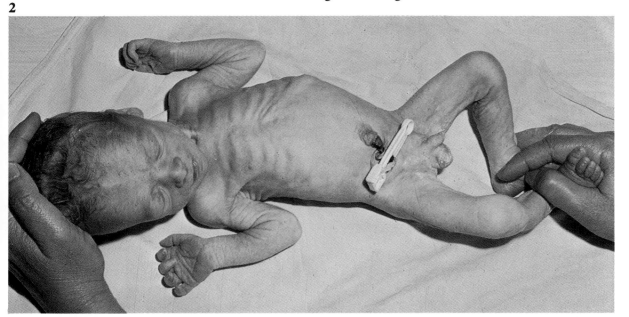

2 "Small-for-dates". Babies who have suffered intrauterine growth retardation are referred to as "small-for dates" or "light-for dates" if the birth-weight is below the 10th centile for gestational age. This baby, of a similar birthweight to the infant in **1**, is 38 weeks gestational age and had suffered chronic intrauterine growth retardation. Note that the skin is less pink, more wrinkled and that the limb posture is more flexed due to increase in tone. It is important to distinguish small-for-dates infants from those who have been chronically growth-retarded. Chronic intrauterine growth retardation causes proportionate restriction of length and head circumference whereas relatively acute intrauterine growth retardation results in a baby who is long and scraggy but who has a normal head circumference.

3 A post-term infant. This baby is 43 weeks gestational age. Note the absence of vernix and the dry cracked and desquamating skin. The umbilical cord is thick and green from meconium staining. No specific treatment for the skin is required. Remember that post-term infants are more prone to pneumonia from meconium aspiration.

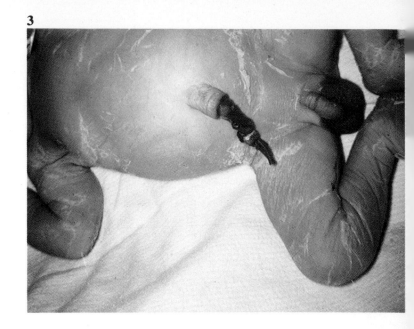

4 "Large-for-dates". A baby weighing more than the 90th centile for gestational age is said to be "large-for-dates" or "heavy-for-dates". This baby who weighed 4.5kg at 38 weeks gestational age is the infant of a diabetic mother (IDM). The IDM is large-for dates due mainly to excess deposition of subcutaneous fat associated with poor maternal metabolic control due to diabetes. IDMs are often hypotonic and are prone to hypoglycaemia, jaundice and the respiratory distress syndrome. There is an increased incidence of major congenital abnormalities (approximately 5%) in IDMs. Note the "frog" position displayed by this baby indicative of hypotonia.

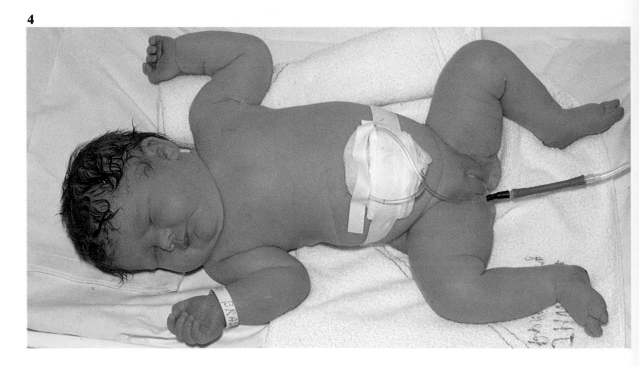

An illustration of the change in a physical characteristic with increasing gestation is demonstrated in the next four illustrations which show the sole of the foot in two pre-term infants, a term infant and a post-term baby.

5

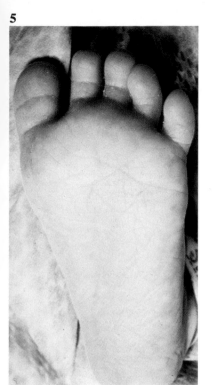

6

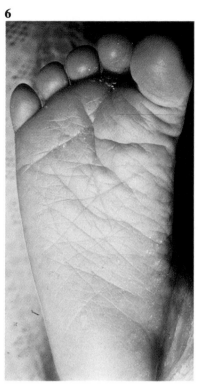

7

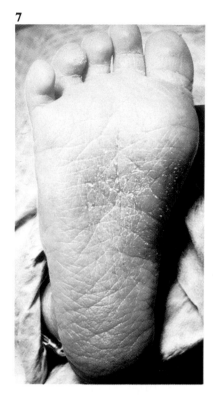

5 The pre-term foot. The sole of this 30-week newborn baby's foot is smooth.

6 The pre-term foot. By 34 weeks creases have started to appear in the anterior one-third of the plantar surface.

7 The term foot. At term the entire plantar area is noticeably creased.

8 The post-term foot. This infant was born at 43 weeks gestational age. Note the excessive creasing on the plantar surface together with dry peeling skin.

8

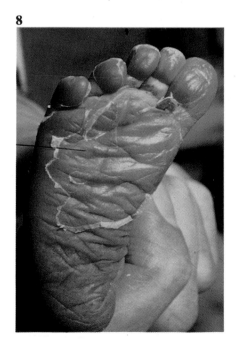

The next group of figures illustrates abnormal posture. This may be temporary and due to the position of the fetus *in utero* (**9**) or more ominous indicating disease as in the hypotonia illustrated in **10**, **11** and **12**.

9

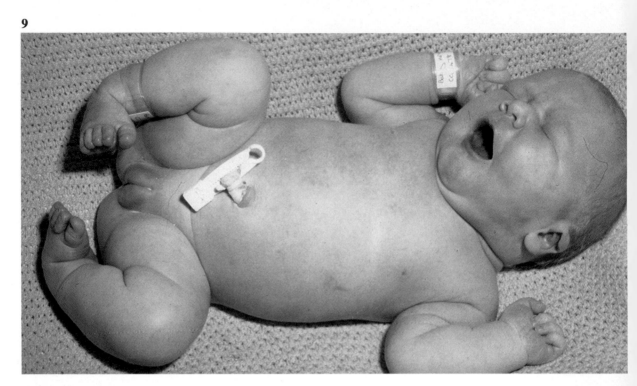

9 Breech posture. Note the un-moulded head, flexed legs and oedema of the left leg and foot in this baby who was a full-term breech delivery with flexed knees.

10

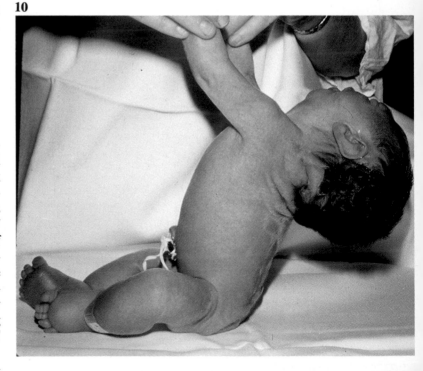

10 Hypotonia. Most term new-born infants can maintain the head in the same plane as the trunk when lifted by the arms or ventral-ly suspended. This baby, who has Turner's syndrome (see also **277** to **280**), shows head lag, a sign of hypotonia. Note also the redundant skin folds in the nape of the neck and the puffiness of the dorsum of the feet. There are many causes of hypotonia including prematurity, brain damage and infection.

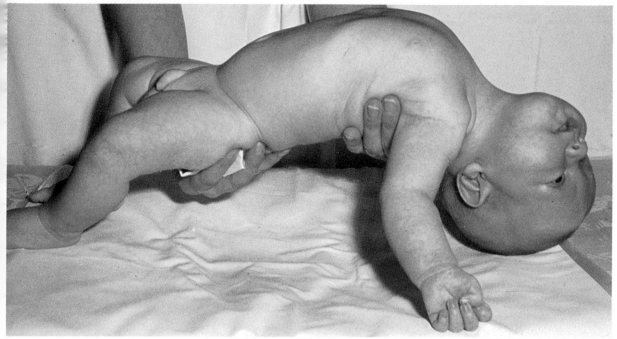

11 Hypotonia. Note the lack of head control on dorsal suspension and the outstretched arms in this baby who has Down's syndrome (see also **269** to **274**).

12

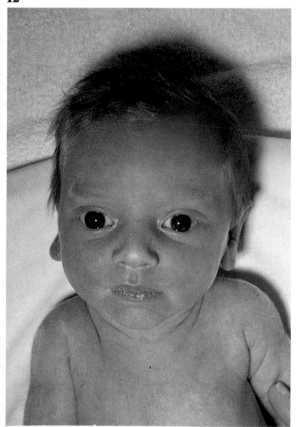

12 Prader–Willi syndrome. This rare congenital syndrome presents with hypotonia in the neonatal period and a characteristic history of feeding difficulty which may result in failure to thrive. This baby shows the characteristic facies of the Prader–Willi syndrome. Such infants grow up to become short, obese adults with mental retardation and hypogenitalism.

13 Prader–Willi syndrome. This figure shows the hand of the baby in **12.** Note the single palmar crease and short fingers. A single palmar crease is commonly found in certain syndromes (see **271**) but may also be an isolated observation in an otherwise normal individual.

13

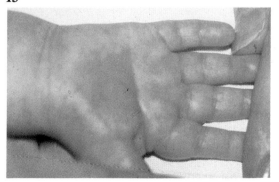

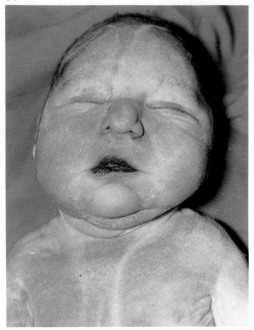

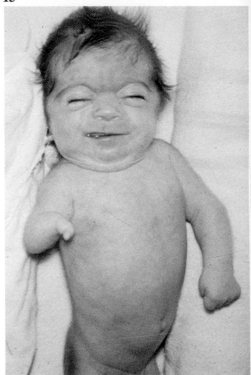

14 Potter's syndrome. This figure shows the head of a fresh stillborn infant suffering from Potter's syndrome. In Potter's syndrome there is renal agenesis or severe renal hypoplasia with resulting oligohydramnios. The babies are small-for-dates and have hypertelorism with lowset, malformed ears. The legs are often malformed with talipes and congenital dislocation of the hips due to pressure deformity from the oligohydramnios. Those who are born alive die in the early neonatal period due to hypoplasia of the lungs or less commonly from renal failure.

15 Cornelia de Lange syndrome. These infants are diagnosed in the neonatal period by recognition of characteristic clinical features: coarse, mop-like hair, eyebrows that meet in the mid-line, a large upper lip and micrognathia. The extremities are characteristically short and pointed. Most infants with Cornelia de Lange syndrome have early feeding difficulties and subsequently show growth failure and severe mental retardation.

16

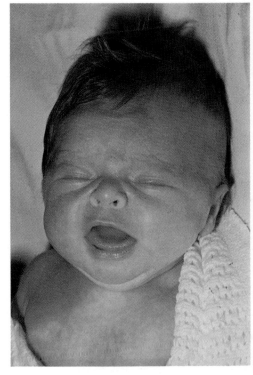

16 Hypothyroidism. Newborn infants with hypothyroidism do not usually have abnormal signs on physical inspection. The characteristic features of cretinism develop in the early weeks and months of life. This infant aged 6 weeks shows features suggestive of cretinism: a snub nose and a large tongue. Hypothyroidism is most commonly diagnosed in the neonatal period as a result of population screening but should always be considered in newborn infants with prolonged jaundice or constipation.

17

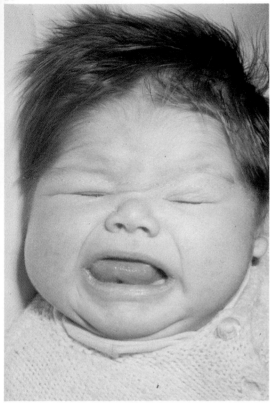

18

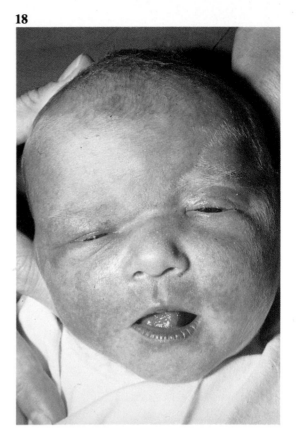

17 Hypothyroidism. This figure shows the infant in **16** at the age of 12 weeks. The facial stigmata of cretinism are now apparent: coarse features and a large tongue.

19

18 and 19 Hemihypertrophy. In this rare condition one side of the body is larger than the other. The aetiology is unknown. Hemihypertrophy may involve the face, arms, trunk and legs or may spare part of the body. Patients with hemihypertrophy have an increased incidence of malignant tumours, particularly Wilm's tumour. It is important but not easy to distinguish hemihypertrophy from hemihypotrophy which is seen for example in Silver–Russell syndrome. In **19** the patient is aged six months and the asymmetry is more clinically obvious.

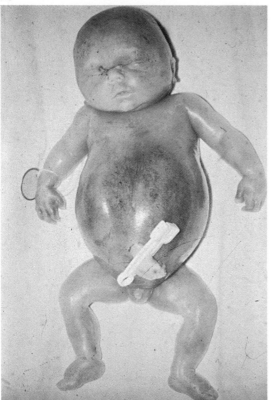

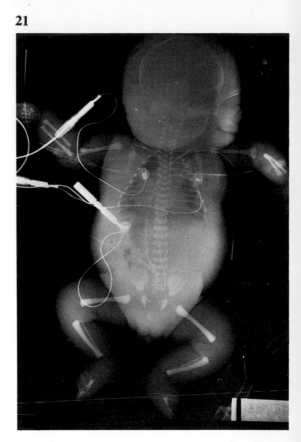

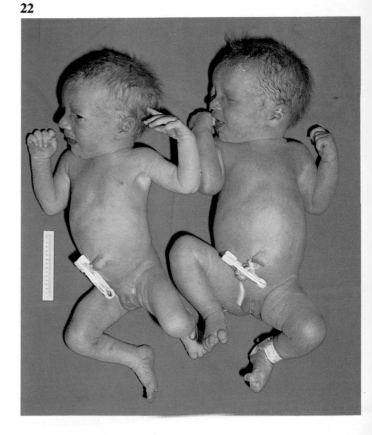

20 Hydrops fetalis results from severe right-sided heart failure *in utero* leading to gross fetal oedema. The commonest cause is severe haemolytic disease usually due to rhesus incompatibility. Note the gross swelling of all parts of the baby and the shiny appearance of the skin. The blue colouration of the abdomen is due to massive hepatic enlargement.

21 Hydrops fetalis. This figure shows the whole body radiograph of an infant with severe hydrops fetalis. Note the increased soft tissue shadowing due to oedema and cardiac enlargement.

22 and 23 Twin-to-twin transfusion: polycythaemia and anaemia. This condition results from abnormal placentation in identical twins in which there is an arterio-venous fistula resulting in one twin becoming polycythaemic and the other anaemic. This figure shows a mild degree of twin-to-twin transfusion in which the twin on the right is pinker than the one on the left: compare the colour of the arms. **23** shows a more striking example of the polycythaemic and anaemic twins. It is important to appreciate that morbidity is more common in the polycythaemic infant who may need a partial exchange transfusion to reduce blood viscosity.

23

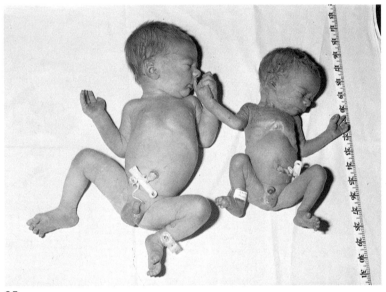

24

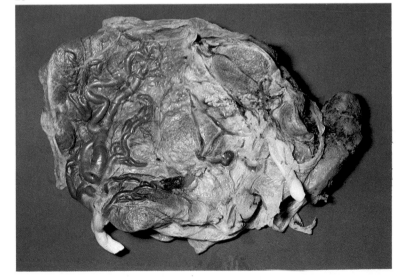

24 Twin-to-twin transfusion: intrauterine growth retardation. The reduction in blood supply to the donor twin can result in intrauterine growth retardation as seen in the twin on the right in this figure.

25

25 Twin-to-twin transfusion: the placentae. This figure shows the placentae of identical twins who had twin-to-twin transfusion. Note the engorged placenta on the left and the pale placenta on the right.

26 and 27 Conjoined twins. This is a rare congenital malformation. In the example shown the babies are joined at the chest and were stillborn. In **27** the single heart shared by both twins is demonstrated at necropsy.

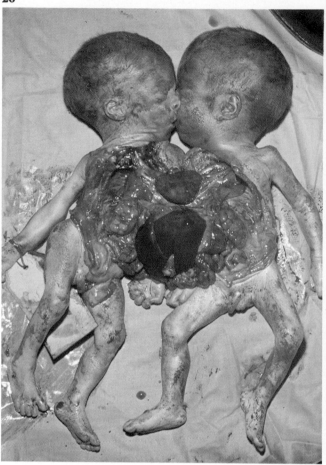

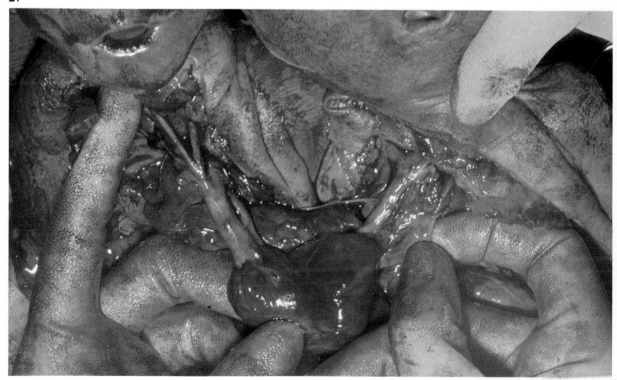

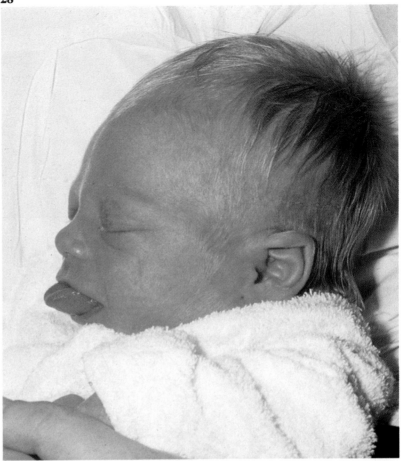

28

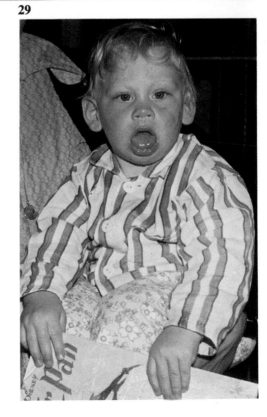

29

28 and 29 Beckwith–Weidemann syndrome. In this anomaly the baby is large-for-dates, has macroglossia, coarse features and hairy ears all of which are seen in this illustration. There is also organomegaly and exomphalos which may result in the baby presenting initially as a surgical problem. Infants with Beckwith–Weidemann syndrome are also prone to hypoglycaemia in the neonatal period. **29** shows the same child as the infant in **28** at the age of 2 years.

2 The head and neck

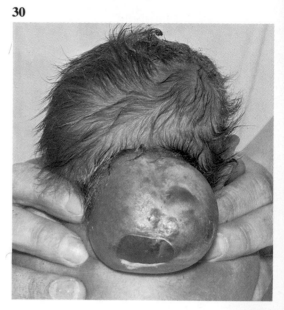

30 and 31 Encephalocoele. Encephalocoeles result from failure of the neuroectodermal axis to develop normally, resulting in congenital bony defects of the skull with protrusion of the meninges which often contain neural tissue. They are most common in the occipital area as shown here. Prognosis is best if the rest of the skull is anatomically normal and no neural tissue has herniated. **31** illustrates the gross hypotonia manifested by the baby seen in **30**.

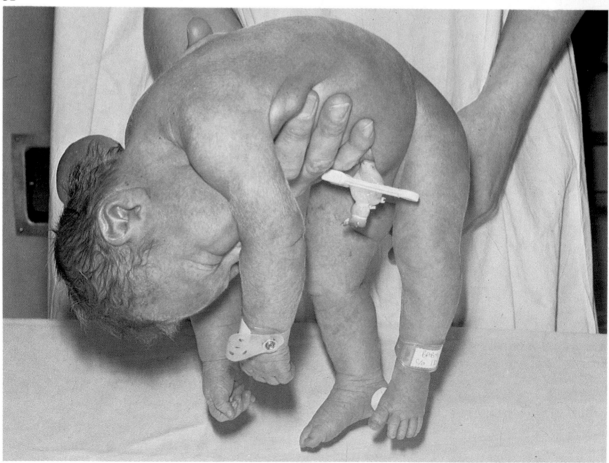

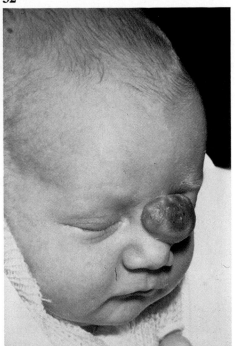

32

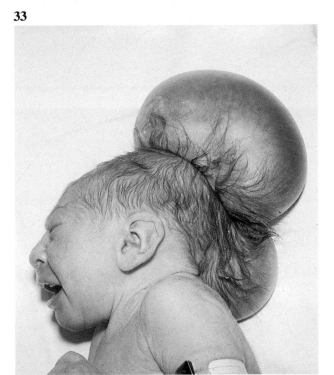

33

32 Encephalocoele. It is important to remember that encephalocoeles may occur at any point in the midline of the skull. Here the encephalocoele protrudes from the base of the nose. It is important to differentiate this lesion from a nasal dermoid.

33 Encephalocoele. This huge encephalocoele arises from the parieto-occipital region and is associated with microcephaly (see also **42**).

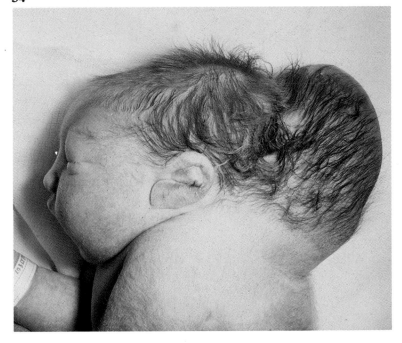

34

34 Encephalocoele/cervical meningocoele. This lesion involves both the occipital region of the skull and cervical spine and is thus both an occipital encephalocoele and a cervical meningocoele. When cervical meningocoele occurs on its own it is unusual for there to be a neurological defect.

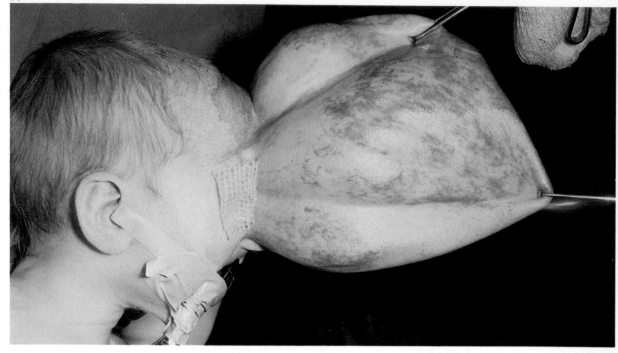

35 Fronto-ethmoid encephalocoele.
Fronto-ethmoid encephalocoeles are rare.
They are characteristically huge and contain much of the frontal cortex and are consequently associated with a poor prognosis.

36

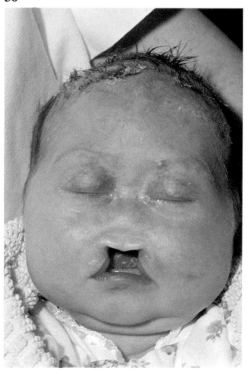

36 and 37 Holoprosencephaly results from maldevelopment of the forebrain (prosencephalon). This may occur as an isolated anomaly or in conjunction with chromosomal abnormality, particularly trisomy 13 (Patau's syndrome, see **281** to **284**). Note the characteristic facial features: cleft lip and palate and narrow-set eyes. Developmental retardation results. A computerized axial tomography (CAT) scan (**37**) shows the characteristic finding in holoprosencephaly: absence of the forebrain with fusion of the lateral ventricles.

37

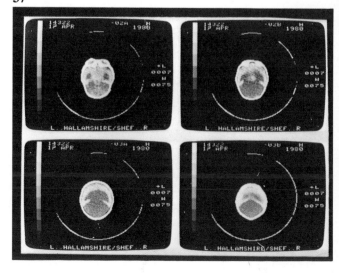

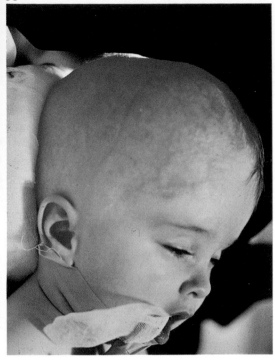

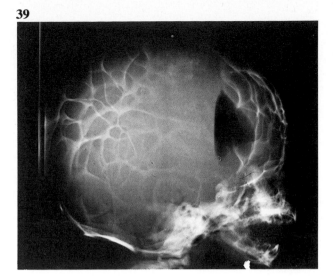

39 Lacunar skull. This radiograph shows a lacunar skull which results from a defect in the formation of membranous bone. The lacunar skull is often associated with hydrocephalus as seen here in an air ventriculogram. The radiological abnormality in the skull disappears with time.

38 Hydranencephaly. In hydranencephaly there is failure of development of the cerebrum with resulting gross dilatation of the ventricles. In this figure the baby's head is illuminated from behind and lights up like an electric bulb. The infant may show abnormal neurological signs from birth and subsequently has poor head growth. Prognosis is poor.

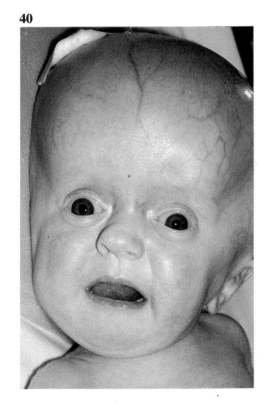

40 and 41 Hydrocephaly results from a block to the drainage of cerebro-spinal fluid which accumulates in the ventricular system under increased pressure resulting in expansion of the skull. Note the large head, distended scalp veins and "sunset" eyes. Hydrocephalus may be idiopathic or secondary to a variety of conditions including spina bifida, meningitis and intraventricular haemorrhage. The diagnosis may be suspected by abnormally rapid head growth and confirmed by ultrasonic or CAT scan investigation. Treatment is most commonly by surgical drainage via a ventriculo-atrial or ventriculo-peritoneal shunt. A valuable clinical diagnostic aid to the diagnosis of hydrocephaly is transillumination of the skull in a dark room (**41**). The accumulation of cerebro-spinal fluid causes thinning of the cerebral mantle and brilliant transillumination may result as shown here.

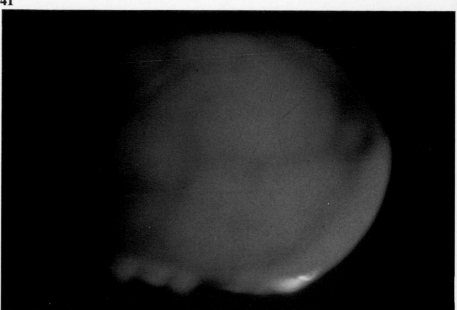

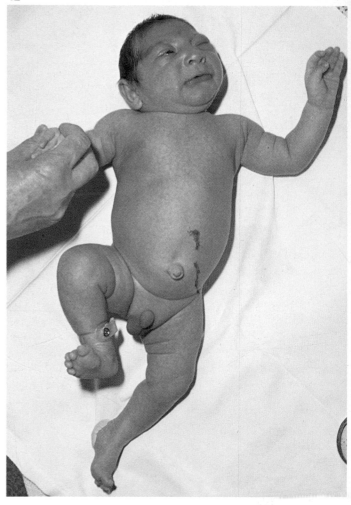

42 Microcephaly may be idiopathic or acquired as a result of intrauterine pathology such as congenital rubella (see **304** to **307**). Microcephaly may also result from serious perinatal brain injury in which case the infant is born with a normal head circumference but the brain fails to grow normally after birth. Severe physical and mental retardation may follow but a minority of infants with microcephaly are neurologically normal.

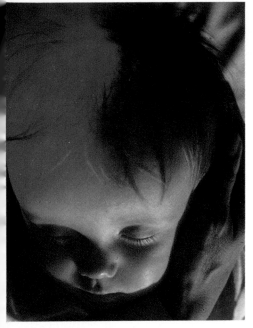

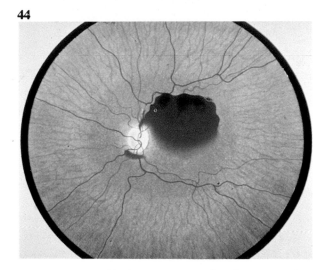

44 Subdural effusion: the optic fundus. In a subdural haemorrhage blood may track through the subdural space along the optic nerve and be visible on fundoscopy as seen here.

43 Subdural effusion. This infant shows increased transillumination unilaterally due to a subdural effusion. Subdural effusion may result from birth trauma or occur as a result of meningitis. The infant presents with generalized irritability, fits and abnormal neurological signs due to raised intracranial pressure.

45 Subdural effusion: cerebral angiogram. Subdural effusion may present in the neonatal period or in later infancy when hydrocephalus may be mimicked. In this figure the cerebral angiogram on the right shows displacement of the blood vessels from the vault of the skull. On the left, air, which has been introduced subdurally following the tapping of the effusion, gives an indication of the size.

45

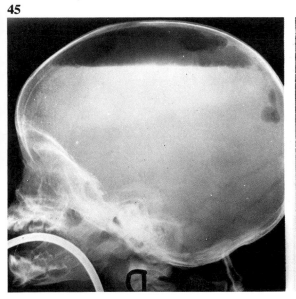 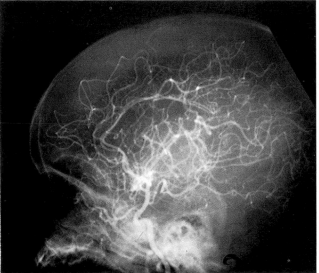

Craniosynostosis results from the premature fusion of one or more of the skull sutures. It is usually suspected because of an abnormal head shape and can be confirmed by radiological examination. Characteristic head shapes result from premature fusion of different skull sutures and are illustrated in the figures overleaf.

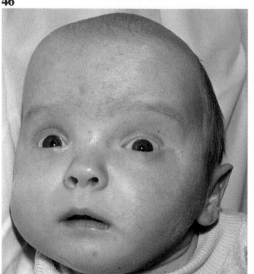

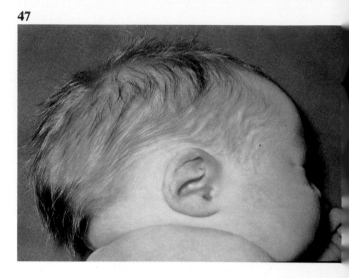

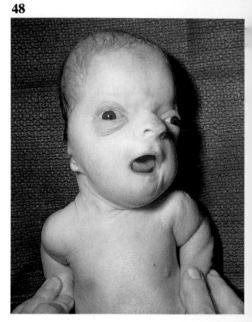

46 Turricephaly. In this patient the head is narrow in the biparietal diameter and domed. Surgery may be of benefit if performed when the infant is under 1 year old.

47 Scaphocephaly. This variant of craniosynostosis is caused by premature fusion of the sagittal suture resulting in a long narrow head. No other problems are usually associated. Scaphocephaly may also be seen as a transient phenomenon lasting up to 1 year in infants born pre-term where there is moulding of the skull from the baby lying on its side.

48 Acrocephaly. This is an example of craniosynostosis caused by premature fusion of the coronal sutures. Note not only the abnormal head shape but also the marked exopthalmos. Surgical treatment is essential.

Craniofacial dysostosis
= Crouzon's dis

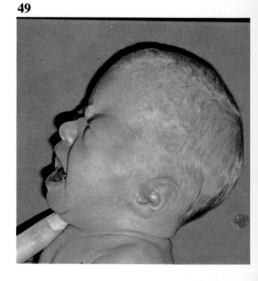

49 Craniofacial dysostosis is also known as Crouzon's disease and is a dominantly inherited condition in which the sutures at the base of the skull fuse prematurely resulting in a brachycephalic skull, proptosis, protrusion of the mandible and occasional hypertelorism.

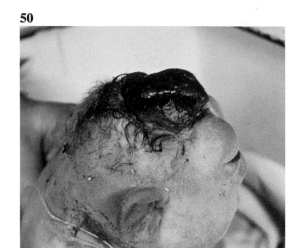

50 Anencephaly. This lethal malformation results from absence of the skull vault and malformation of the underlying brain. The infant may be stillborn. Anencephaly should be suspected in any case of unexplained polyhydramnios and is one of the causes of a raised serum and amniotic alphafetoprotein.

51 Intraventricular haemorrhage (IVH) occurs characteristically in pre-term infants, usually those who have suffered hypoxia or acidosis. It may also occur rarely in full-term infants. Intraventricular haemorrhage varies in severity and the pathological specimen illustrated here shows a grade IV haemorrhage which is usually lethal. Infants who survive a major intraventricular haemorrhage may subsequently develop cerebral palsy and/or hydrocephalus due to blockage of the ventricular drainage system.

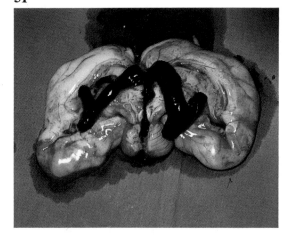

52 Intraventricular haemorrhage: CAT scan. This figure shows two CAT scans taken of an infant 2 weeks apart. On the left the dilated ventricles are seen to be filled with blood (white), which has extended into the brain substance. On the right much of the blood has been resorbed but the ventricles are grossly dilated indicating the development of hydrocephalus.

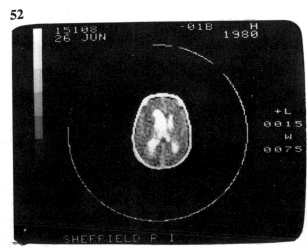
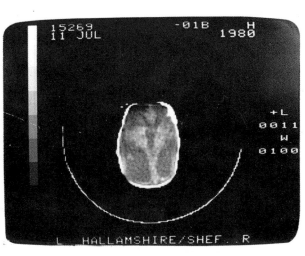

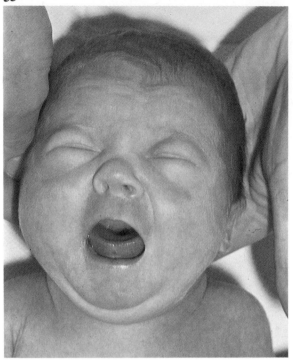

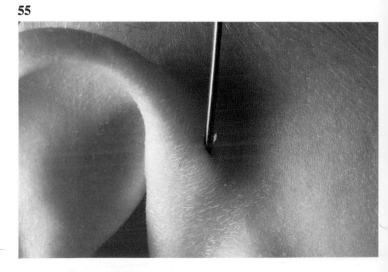

53 Neonatal oedema. Oedema in the newborn can result from fluid overload for any reason but is most commonly seen in cardiac failure. The signs of oedema in the newborn are most characteristically seen around the eyes as shown here and as puffiness on the dorsum of the feet.

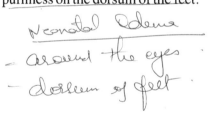

Neonatal Oedema
- around the eyes
- dorsum of feet

54 Congenital nephrotic syndrome. This baby has gross generalized oedema which was associated with proteinuria and hypoproteinaemia. The condition is exceedingly rare. The infant usually develops early renal failure and the prognosis is poor.

55

55 Preauricular sinus. This is a small pit in the skin shown by the probe immediately in front of the helix of the ear. A preauricular sinus may be blind or may communicate with the internal ear or the brain. Chronic infection is occasionally a problem, and may be dangerous if the sinus communicates with the central nervous system.

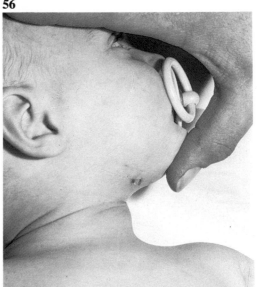

56 Branchial sinus. A branchial sinus may occur anywhere between the mastoid and the sternum along the line of the sternomastoid muscle. The sinus shown here appears as a small hole in the submandibular region. These sinuses may communicate with deeper structures and discharge purulent material. Treatment is surgical and requires dissection of the entire sinus tract.

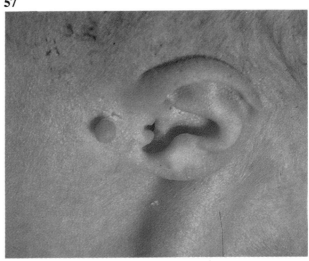

57 Accessory auricle. This is an asymptomatic pedunculated skin tag which is seen most commonly at the junction of the maxillary and mandibular processes of the first branchial arch. Surgical treatment is given for cosmetic reasons.

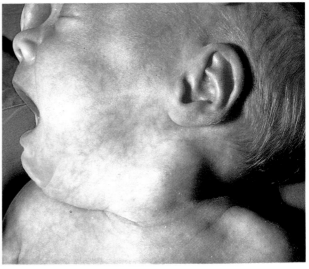

58 Sternomastoid tumour. This is a lump appearing in the sternomastoid muscle which usually becomes clinically apparent in the second week of life. It may enlarge for several weeks before resolving spontaneously. A sternomastoid tumour may result in torticollis. Most cases are idiopathic, but some are due to bruising within the sternomastoid muscle.

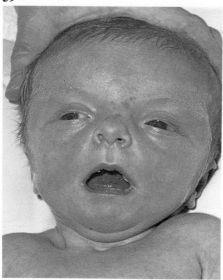

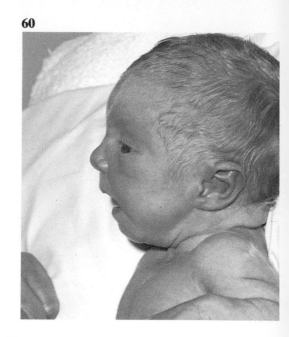

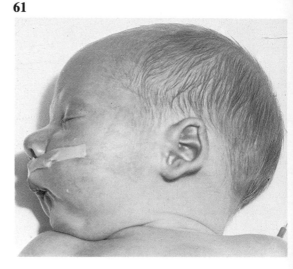

The next four figures illustrate babies with small jaws but for different reasons.

59 and 60 Choanal atresia and micrognathia. Choanal atresia results from blockage of one or both nasal septa and may present shortly after birth with cyanosis which is relieved when the infant cries. Unilateral choanal atresia may present later in life with inability to breath through one side of the nose. Note the blocked right nostril and micrognathia in this case. Diagnosis of choanal atresia is made by inability to pass a nasogastric tube. **60** is a lateral view of the same infant seen in **59** and shows the micrognathia more clearly.

61 Pierre–Robin syndrome. This is characterized by micrognathia, a posterior cleft palate and a protruding tongue. The infant is prone to cyanotic attacks caused by the tongue falling back and obstructing the posterior oropharynx. The infant should be nursed prone. With time the micrognathia improves and surgery is seldom required.

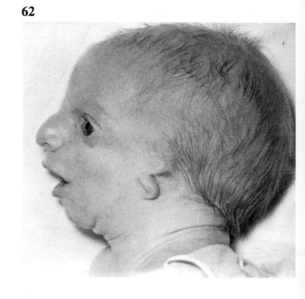

62 Seckel dwarf. Seckel dwarfs are also known as "bird-headed" dwarfs and are born small-for-dates with a characteristic microcephaly, premature synostosis, large eyes, beaked nose, lowset ears and micrognathia. Other congenital defects may be present. Postnatal growth is extremely retarded and some degree of mental retardation may also be present.

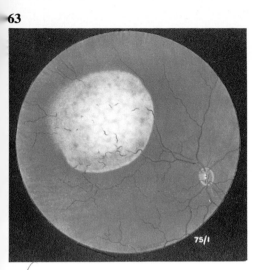

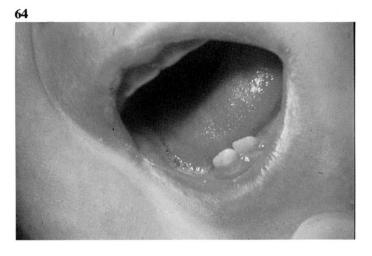

63 Retinoblastoma. This rare tumour, which often runs in families, may present at birth. The classical clinical sign is an opaque or a white pupil but some present with a squint or glaucoma. Retinoblastoma tends to spread along the optic nerve or distally via the choroid. Prognosis is variable and depends upon early diagnosis.

64 Congenital tooth. These may be present at birth or erupt in the first month of life. They are nearly always very loose and thus easy to extract.

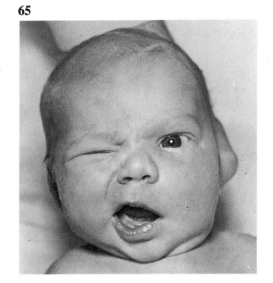

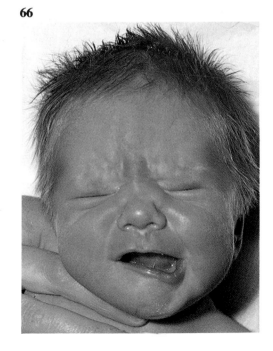

65 and 66 Facial palsy is a fairly common condition in the newborn due to pressure on the facial nerve distal to the stylomastoid foramen usually caused by forceps application during delivery. On the affected right side the baby is unable to close the eye or contract the lower facial muscles. The condition is usually self-limiting. In **66** the baby shows a milder variant in which there is weakness of the muscles controlling movement of the mouth but not those of the upper face. This is known as the "asymmetric crying facies".

67 Cleft lip. Bilateral cleft lip results from failure of fusion of the nasomedial or intermaxillary process with the maxillary process. Cleft lip may be unilateral or bilateral and is often associated with cleft palate. It is important to arrange immediate referral to a surgeon expert in the treatment of cleft lip and palate since he will be able to do much to restore parental morale by showing them photographs of patients with an excellent cosmetic result following treatment.

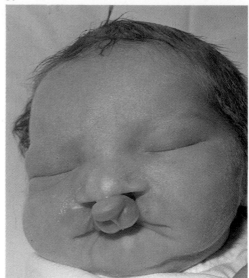

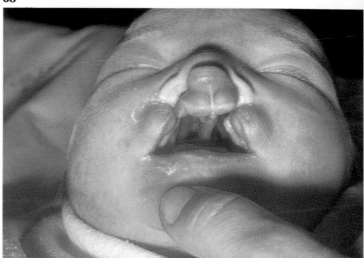

68 Cleft palate. This figure is of the same infant as seen in **67** showing a bilateral cleft palate.

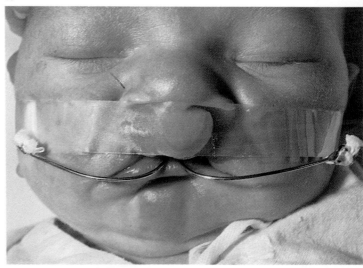

69 Cleft lip and palate with orthodontic plate. This figure illustrates one mode of treatment available which is to provide an orthodontic plate that covers the cleft palate thus enabling the child to feed normally until surgical correction is undertaken.

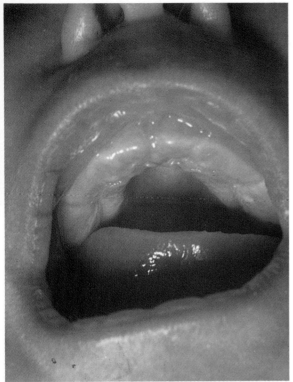

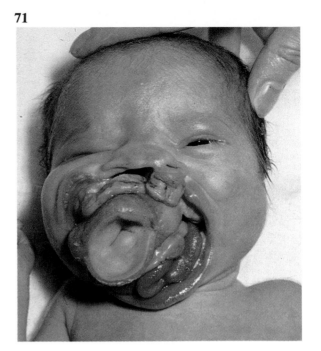

71 Gross cleft lip and palate. This infant seems to display an extreme variant of cleft lip and palate. The lower lip is intact, but there is extensive bilateral upper cleft with rotation of the hard and soft palate. In addition there is a posterior cleft of the hard palate. The tongue is laterally displaced and cleft. The appearance simulates an orifice within an orifice.

70 Posterior cleft palate. This may occur in the absence of a cleft lip. Feeding difficulties can ensue with regurgitation of milk into the nasopharynx. The infant may have difficulty sucking efficiently and may thus present as a feeding problem.

72 Ranula is a mucous cyst of one of the sublingual salivary glands and is apparent as a smooth, soft, grey swelling in the floor of the mouth. Treatment is by surgical eventration.

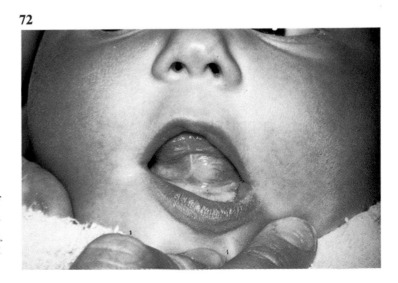

73 Anophthalmia. This rare condition may be unilateral or bilateral and may occur as an isolated defect or in association with genetic disorders such as trisomy 13 (Patau's syndrome – see **281** to **284**). The eye may be totally absent or very small (microphthalmia).

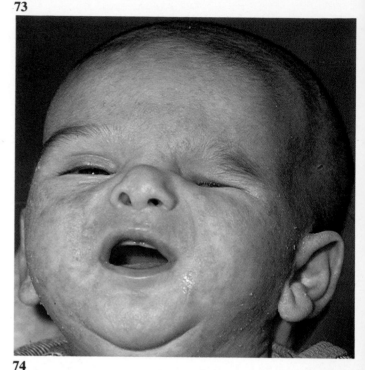

74 Subconjunctival haemorrhage. A linear or lunar haemorrhage is often seen to the side of the iris immediately after delivery and is not related to perinatal trauma. Subconjunctival haemorrhage is self-limiting and does not require treatment.

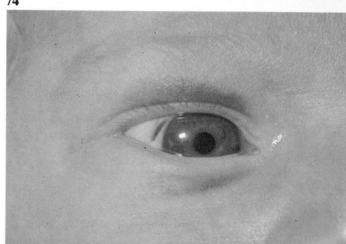

75 Conjunctivitis. Mild conjunctivitis (sticky eye) is often seen in the newborn and may be caused by staphylococci, pneumococci or a virus. Conjunctivitis may be gross as in the case illustrated here which was due to gonococcal ophthalmia. Gonococcal ophthalmia usually presents within the first 24 hours of life and may lead to systemic infection. In all cases of conjunctivitis bacteriological investigation is indicated and both eyes must be treated. In many countries silver nitrate or other solutions are administered to the eyes prophylactically, but the treatment may cause severe chemical conjunctivitis and is not recommended.

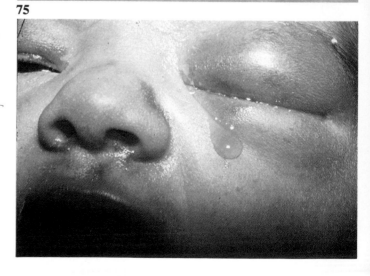

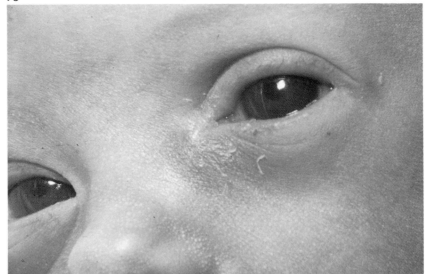

76 Acute dacrocystitis. This is an infection of the nasolacrimal duct and follows duct blockage. In mild cases antibiotic therapy combined with gentle massage of the duct may suffice, in more serious cases it is necessary to probe the duct under general anaesthetic.

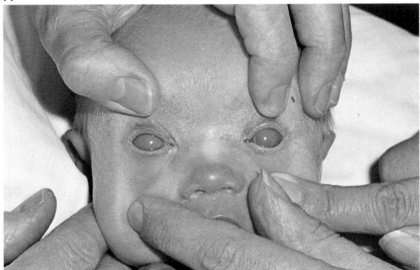

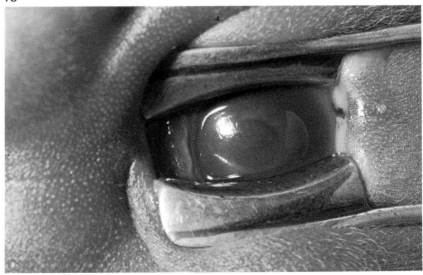

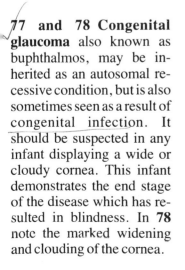

77 and 78 Congenital glaucoma also known as buphthalmos, may be inherited as an autosomal recessive condition, but is also sometimes seen as a result of congenital infection. It should be suspected in any infant displaying a wide or cloudy cornea. This infant demonstrates the end stage of the disease which has resulted in blindness. In **78** note the marked widening and clouding of the cornea.

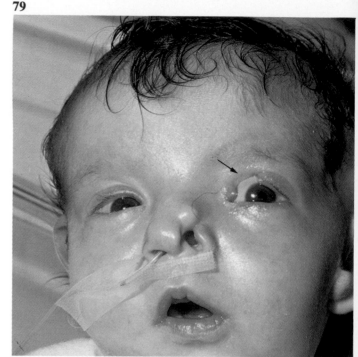

79 Coloboma of eyelid: Goldenhar's syndrome. A coloboma is a skin defect of the eyelid and in this case affects the supero-medial margin of the left upper eyelid. Colobomata are present in many syndromes, both genetic and sporadic. This baby also has a deformity of the left nostril, unequal mandibular development and a hemivertebra. This collection of stigmata is known as Goldenhar's syndrome.

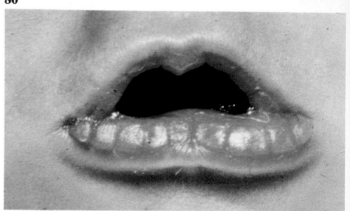

80 Sucking blisters. These superficial lesions are often found on the lips and sometimes on the fingers of newborn infants. They disappear spontaneously shortly after birth.

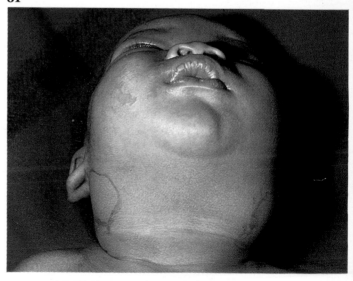

81 Cervical abscess. This infant has bilateral cervical abscesses. This is rare in the neonatal period but can occur secondary to any suppurative condition in the upper airway. It may also result from congenital tuberculosis. Treatment consists of treating the primary cause and draining the abscess.

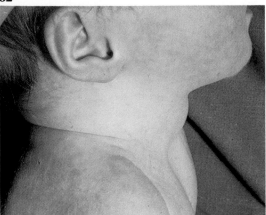

82 Neonatal goitre. Goitre may occur in the newborn due to maternal iodine deficiency, drug ingestion, maternal thyrotoxicosis or inborn errors of thyroxine biosynthesis. Pressure effects on the trachea may result in respiratory distress. Medical treatment depends on whether the infant is hypo- or hyperthyroid.

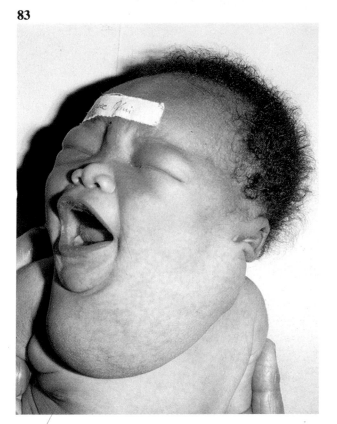

83 and 84 Cystic hygroma. The term cystic hygroma refers to a large lymphangioma. **83** illustrates a large cavernous lymphangioma of the neck. A cystic hygroma may involve any part of the body but characteristically involves the face and upper trunk. Treatment is surgical. **84** illustrates a cystic hygroma of the cheek which transilluminates.

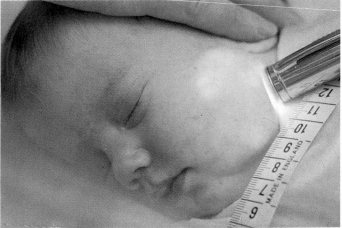

3 The arms and legs

Club foot may be of an equino-varus or calcaneo-valgus variety.

85

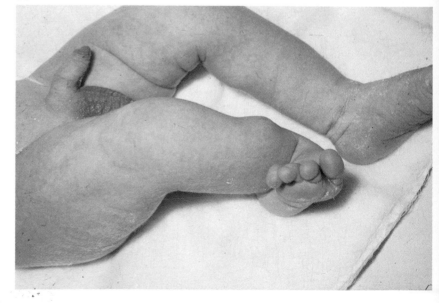

85 Talipes equino-varus. This figure shows an example of talipes equino-varus in which the foot is inverted, plantar flexed and adducted. Both feet are often affected. Orthopaedic advice should be sought at birth. Initial management involves physiotherapy and splinting of the feet. In a minority of cases surgery may subsequently be necessary.

86

86 Talipes calcaneo-valgus. In talipes calcaneo-valgus the foot is everted and dorsiflexed. It may result from abnormal intrauterine posture or be associated with lower motor neurone defects such as spina bifida. Treatment is initially by manipulation and splinting but surgical correction may be necessary.

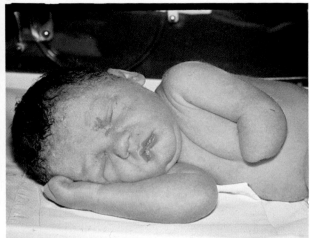

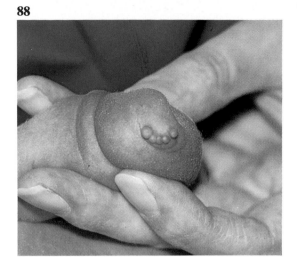

87 and 88 Intrauterine amputation occurs rarely and usually involves the distal part of the limb. The cause is unknown although amniotic bands interfering with the development of the embryonic limbs have been suggested to be responsible. The infant is otherwise normal. **88** shows the forearm end on of the baby shown in **87**. Note the rudimentary digits growing from the foreshortened forearm.

89

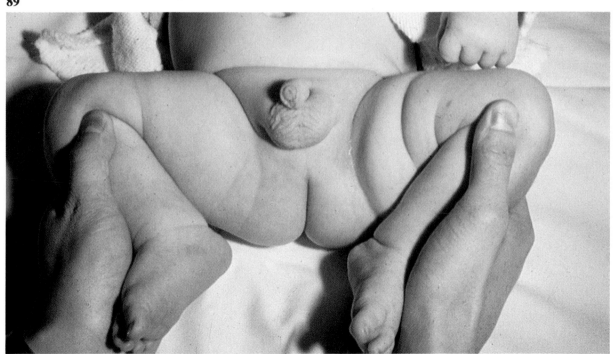

89 Congenital dislocation of the hip (CDH) occurs more frequently in girls and is an uncommon but clinically very important lesion with an incidence of 4 to 7 per 1000 births. CDH may be suspected clinically by asymmetry of the skin creases in the groins as seen here. Physical examination shows limited abduction of the affected left side.

90 and 91 Congenital dislocation of the hip: radiographs. In **90** the radiograph of the pelvis shows a shallow acetabulum on the affected left side associated with poor development of the upper femoral epiphysis. Neonatal treatment of CDH involves splinting the legs in flexion and abduction which may be achieved most simply by the use of a double nappy but more commonly involves a frog splint. In **91** the radiograph shows a patient who has worn a splint for several months and in whom there is improvement of the alignment of the upper femoral epiphysis to the acetabulum.

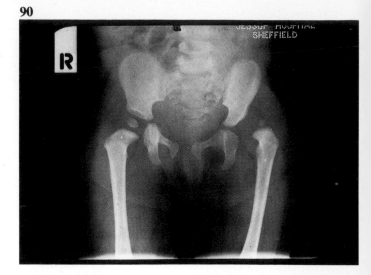

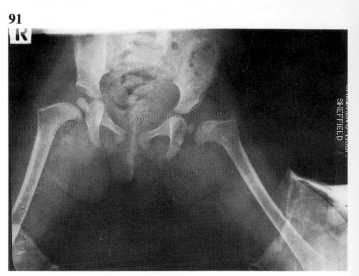

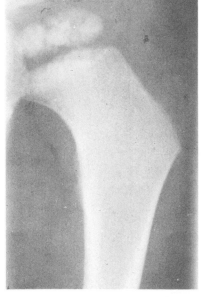

92 Epiphyseal dysplasia. This radiograph demonstrates an irregular fragmented epiphysis of the femoral head. This finding may be seen in untreated CDH and is commonly seen in neonatal hypothyroidism (see **16** and **17**).

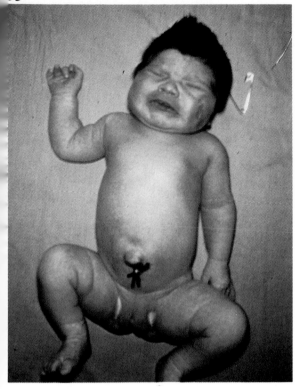

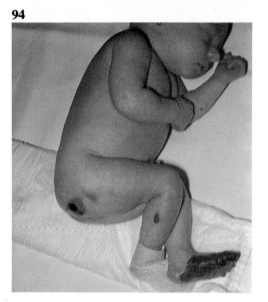

93 Erb's palsy usually results from a traumatic delivery in which the neck has been hyper-extended and the brachial plexus damaged particularly that part involving spinal nerve roots C_3, C_4 and C_5. Clinically the infant presents with a paralysed arm which is held in the extended position with dorsiflexion of the wrist. Occasionally ipsilateral paralysis of the diaphragm may occur.

94 and 95 Gangrene of the buttock and foot. Umbilical arterial catheterization may be associated with thrombotic complications (see also **368**). In this patient intra-arterial injection of alkali was followed by gangrene of the right buttock and outer aspect of the right calf. This complication resulted from spasm and thrombosis of the internal obturator artery which supplies the muscles of the buttock and the arteries of the left foot. The risks associated with umbilical arterial catheterization must not be underestimated and have led some neonatologists to prefer peripheral arterial catheterization, e.g. of the radial or posterior tibial artery.

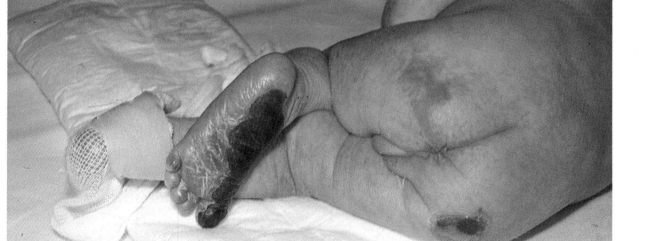

96 and 97 Ulceration of the arm. In **96** a large area of necrosis of the posterior aspect of the left upper arm is seen. This resulted from overtight strapping of the arm to secure a peripheral intravenous infusion. The permanent scarring which resulted from the necrotic area is seen in **97.**

96

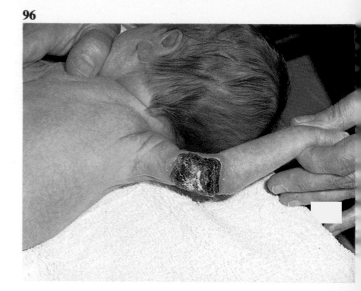

97

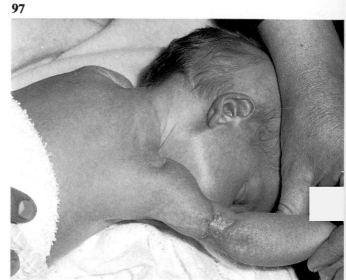

98 Injection of contrast medium. This baby was unfortunate to receive a direct injection of contrast medium *in utero* into the anterior aspect of the left upper arm. The figure shows the severe local reaction that was clinically apparent at birth.

99 Ulceration of the leg. This example of severe third degree ulceration of the antero-medial aspect of the left leg resulted from extravasation of an intravenous infusion containing calcium. Ulceration may follow the subcutaneous leakage of any hypertonic solution but those containing calcium are particularly irritant. The infant subsequently required a skin graft.

99

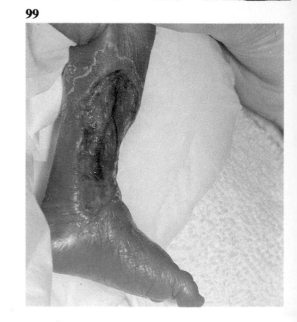

98

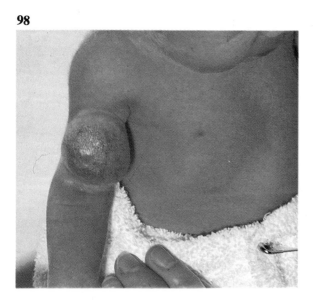

100 Osteomyelitis of the tibia.
Osteomyelitis in the newborn is usually staphylococcal and may be difficult to diagnose due to paucity of clinical signs. Characteristically the infant with osteomyelitis of a limb is reluctant to move the limb spontaneously, but may or may not show signs of being generally unwell. Localized signs include swelling and tenderness of the affected region. Radiological changes occur late and demonstrate cortical destruction and widening of the shaft. Treatment in all cases is with appropriate systemic antibiotic therapy. On occasion surgical drainage may be necessary.

101 Osteomyelitis of the humerus.
This figure shows similar changes to those seen in **100.** It is important to remember that osteomyelitis may be associated with septic arthritis in the newborn.

102 and 103   Rickets is now being diagnosed with increasing frequency as more very small babies survive. Unless the possibility of diagnosing rickets is kept under active clinical review the

(continued overleaf)

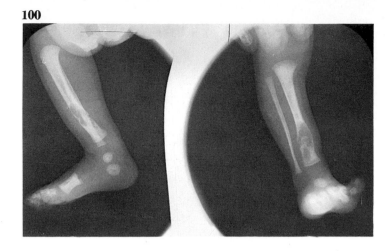

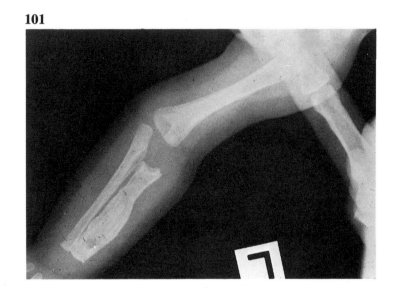

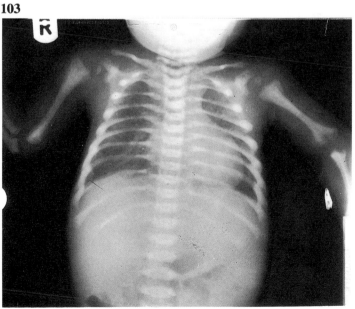

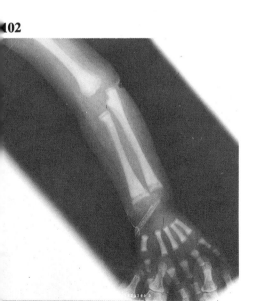

diagnosis may often be made as a co-incidental radiological finding. In **102** note the fraying and ragged appearance of the distal end of the radius and ulna with widening of the joint space. **103** shows a case of rickets that was diagnosed fortuitously by careful examination of the chest radiograph in which thickening of the costochondral junction is well displayed (rickety rosary). Very pre-term infants are vitamin D resistant and supplements of 1000 units of cholecalciferol per day are commonly used in their management.

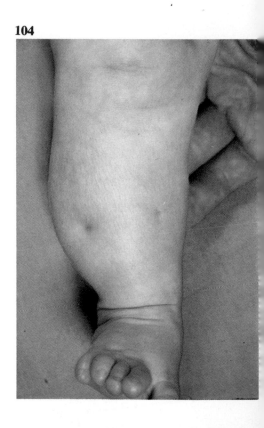

104

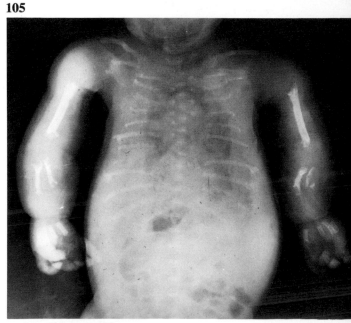

105

104 and 105 Hypophosphatasia is extremely rare and results from an inborn error of deficiency of alkaline phosphatase, resulting in failure of calcification of all bones. A classical physical sign is dimpling over the distal tibia and fibula as seen in **104**. The infant fails to thrive and shows feeding difficulties and general irritability. Other physical and biochemical information suggests rickets but the serum alkaline phosphatase level is low or absent rather than being elevated. **105** shows the gross osteoporosis and flaring of the metaphyseal regions of the long bones in a case of hypophosphatasia.

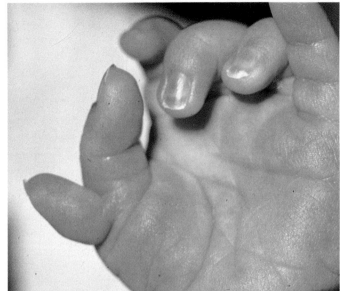

106 Polydactyly may occur as an isolated finding, sometimes inherited dominantly, or may be part of many syndromes. The extra digit usually has no skeletal elements and may be tied off if the base is narrow. Otherwise surgical removal is necessary.

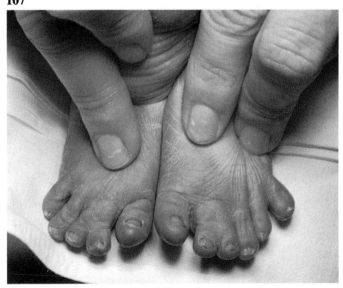

107 Syndactyly is not uncommon and involves the toes more frequently than the fingers. This figure illustrates syndactyly of the second and third toes which may cause parental concern but is of no medical or cosmetic significance. Note also the extra digit on the left foot for which surgical treatment is required.

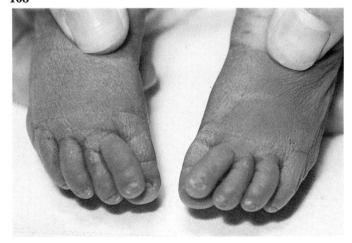

108 Overlapping toes occur commonly, in this case the second and third toes are overlapping the big toe. The condition causes parental concern in the neonatal period, but reassurance is indicated since the abnormality usually becomes less as development continues and does not interfere with locomotion.

109 Radial dysplasia. The clinical signs of radial dysplasia include a shortening of the radial aspect of the forearm with radial displacement of the hand. Varying degrees of dysplasia occur, ranging from complete absence of the radius with major malformation of the radial side of the hand, to normal development of the radius and only minor anomalies of the thumb. In this figure there is absence of the radius and thumb and malformation of the first finger. Radial dysplasia may be associated with congenital heart disease, aplastic anaemia and abnormalities of other parts of the skeleton.

110 Sirenomelia. Infants with sirenomelia may also be known as "mermaid babies". This very rare disorder is characterized by fusion of all or part of the lower limbs and numerous other deformities affecting in particular the kidneys and gastrointestinal tract. It is incompatible with life.

110

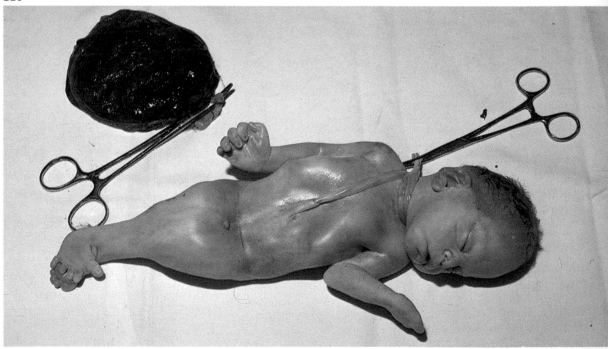

4 The chest

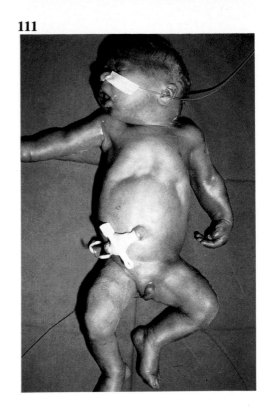

111 Rib recession. Newborn infants often show inter-costal, subcostal and sternal inspiratory recession because of the pliability of the chest wall. This is an important clinical sign which reflects stiffness of the lungs often due to respiratory distress syndrome or other neonatal respiratory problems. This infant was born at 31 weeks gestation with a birthweight of 2.6 kg and was subsequently shown to have the Beckwith–Weidemann syndrome (**28, 29**).

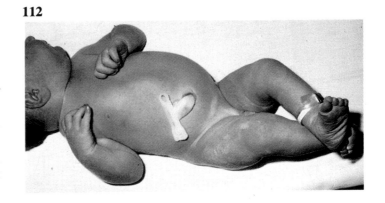

112 Peripheral cyanosis. Cyanosis of the hands and feet is a common clinical finding in normal babies during the first 24 hours of life. It arises from slow peripheral circulation and may be associated with hypothermia. Spontaneous improvement always occurs.

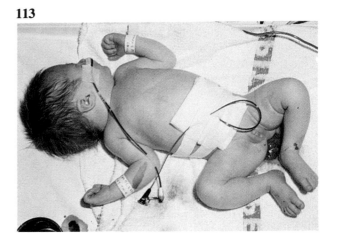

113 Central cyanosis. Cyanosis is commonly observed in the immediate neonatal period but when seen following resuscitation and in the absence of obvious respiratory problems, cyanosis is usually a sign of cardiac disease. In this baby there was also a suspicion of necro-tizing enterocolitis (see **165** to **168**) because of the passage of blood-stained meconium.

114 Hyaline membrane disease. Respiratory distress may be due to a variety of causes, the commonest of which in the pre-term infant is hyaline membrane disease. The baby classically presents with tachypnoea, an expiratory grunt, inspiratory intercostal, subcostal and sternal recession (see **111**) and nasal flaring. Classically the diagnosis of hyaline membrane disease is not made until 4 hours or more after birth to help distinguish the condition from transient tachypnoea of the newborn (see **115**). The chest X-ray shows poor aeration, air bronchogram and a generalized ''ground glass'' appearance of the lung fields.

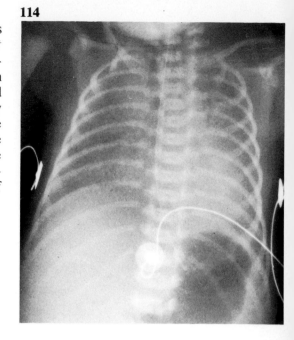

115 Wet lung is the descriptive term used for the radiological features of infants experiencing transient tachypnoea of the newborn. Both titles are descriptive and refer to the problem arising from delayed clearance of lung fluid which is normally expelled partly by the trachea and partly absorbed via the pulmonary lymphatics. Wet lung may occur at all gestational ages and can be easily mistaken for hyaline membrane disease. Important distinguishing features are the earlier onset and speedy spontaneous resolution of wet lung. The radiograph shows changes suggestive of hyaline membrane disease but note particularly fluid in the horizontal fissure on the right (arrow).

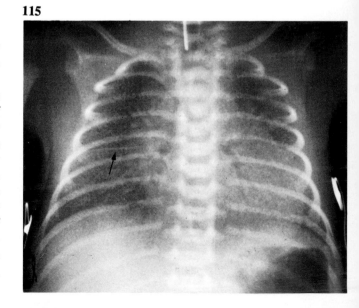

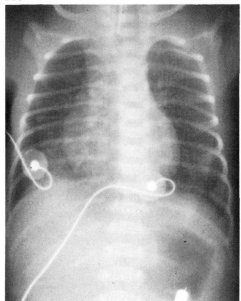

116 Streptococcal pneumonia. Pneumonia due to Group B streptococcal infection must be considered in any baby presenting with symptoms of respiratory distress since this condition is rapidly fatal. Comparison of the radiographic findings in this figure with those in **114** illustrates the similarity of the two conditions.

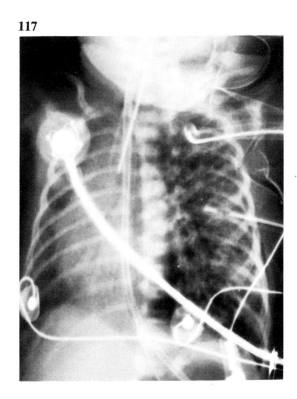

117 Interstitial emphysema. This is caused by widespread rupture of the alveoli resulting in the accumulation of air in the interstitial lung tissue. Interstitial emphysema may complicate hyaline membrane disease and occur during mechanically assisted ventilation or spontaneously. Pneumothorax and pneumomediastinum are complications. In this infant only the left lung is affected and a good recovery followed the selective intubation of the right main bronchus and ventilation of the baby by the right lower lobe alone. Note the two pneumothorax drains present on the left side.

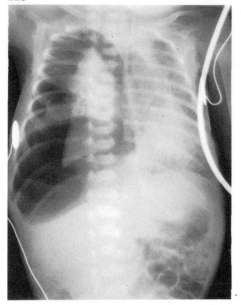

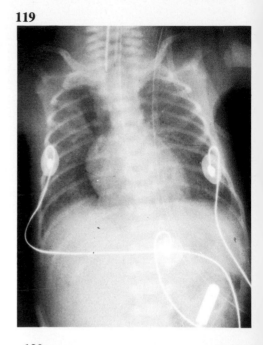

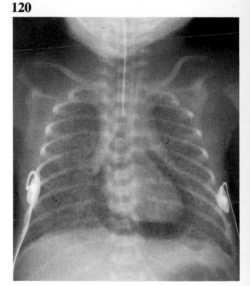

118 Pneumothorax in the newborn may occur spontaneously, or more commonly as a complication of assisted ventilation in pre-term infants. A small pneumothorax may require no active treatment but more commonly pneumothorax is associated with a positive pressure air leak and rapid clinical deterioration due to mediastinal shift and collapse of the lungs. Diagnosis may be made most rapidly by transillumination of the chest wall and confirmed by a radiograph. Treatment involves insertion of a chest drain with rapid symptomatic recovery.

119 Pneumomediastinum. Rupture of alveoli may occur not into the pleural space, but into the mediastinal space with accumulation of air around the heart. A gross pneumomediastinum may be seen on a PA film as shown in this figure, but lesser degrees are only seen in lateral chest radiographs as a bubble between the heart and sternum. Active treatment of a pneumomediastinum is not usually necessary.

120 Pneumopericardium results when alveolar rupture leads to interstitial emphysema and tracking of air along the pulmonary veins into the pericardium. Pneumopericardium may resolve spontaneously òr more rarely result in cardiac tamponade as seen in this figure.

121 Right middle lobe pneumonia. This figure shows the radiograph of an infant with consolidation and collapse of the right middle lobe and hyperinflation of the remainder of the right lung. Bacterial pneumonia may result from a variety of organisms but Group B Streptococci, *Staphylococcus aureus* and Coliforms are most commonly involved.

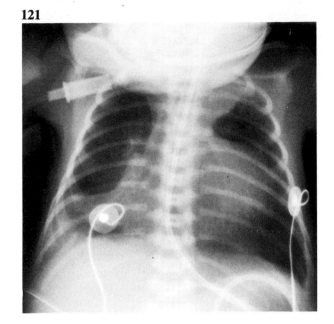

122 Pulmonary haemorrhage. Massive pulmonary haemorrhage is a rare but usually lethal condition affecting most commonly small-for-dates babies (see **2**). It is often associated with cold injury of the newborn and is seen more rarely than hitherto because of care taken to keep small infants warm. The presenting clinical sign is the coughing of frothy, blood-stained mucus or the aspiration of blood-stained liquid from the trachea. Auscultation reveals widespread fine crepitations which may not be heard if the infant is receiving positive pressure ventilation. Massive pulmonary haemorrhage may be associated with a bleeding diathesis or occur independently. The chest radiograph may resemble hyaline membrane disease (**114**) or massive consolidation as seen in this figure.

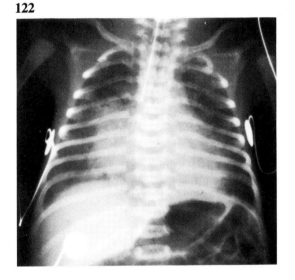

123 Bronchopulmonary dysplasia (BPD, not to be confused with biparietal diameter) occurs in infants who have received prolonged oxygen therapy usually together with mechanical ventilation. The diagnosis is made in an infant aged 1 week or more who shows signs of chronic respiratory insufficiency following treatment for hyaline membrane disease. The radiograph shows a honeycomb picture in the lung fields. Approximately one-third of babies with BPD die of respiratory failure, one-third develop chronic pulmonary disease and one-third recover.

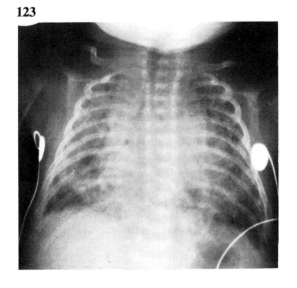

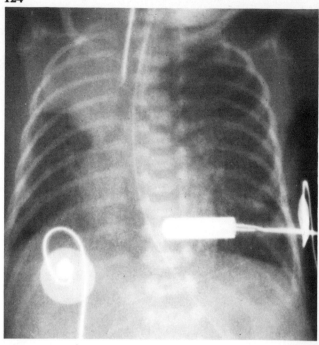

124 Atelectasis of the right upper lobe. Atelectasis is commonly seen in babies receiving positive pressure ventilation. As a result of being nursed prone secretions may accumulate in the right upper lobe bronchus and cause collapse. The radiograph shows an opacity in the right upper zone which extends to the chest wall and must not be confused with the thymus. Treatment is by physiotherapy.

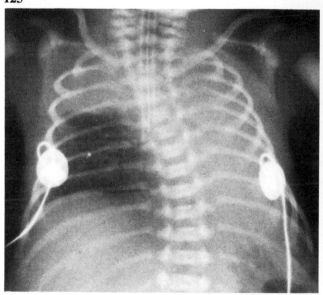

125 Misplaced endotracheal tube. In this baby the endotracheal tube has been passed too far into the right main bronchus with resulting atelectasis of the left lung and right upper lobe. It is easy to avoid passing the endotracheal tube too far by palpating the sternal notch and feeling for the tip of the tube. When the tube tip can be felt at the sternal notch it lies halfway down the trachea.

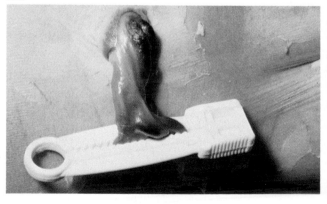

126 Meconium staining of the umbilical cord. This meconium stained umbilical cord is an important physical sign indicating that the fetus has passed meconium *in utero* and is at risk of meconium aspiration.

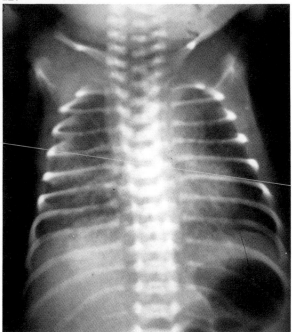

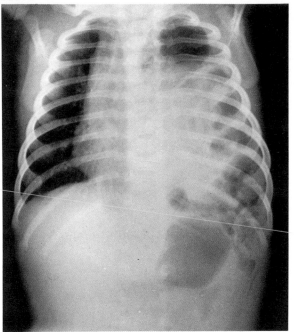

127 Meconium aspiration. If the infant aspirates meconium stained liquor due to making respiratory effort during delivery severe respiratory distress can result. Meconium aspiration is more common in term and post-term infants and may cause a severe chemical pneumonia. The radiological changes vary from lobar consolidation to widespread opacities involving both lung fields in the severest cases.

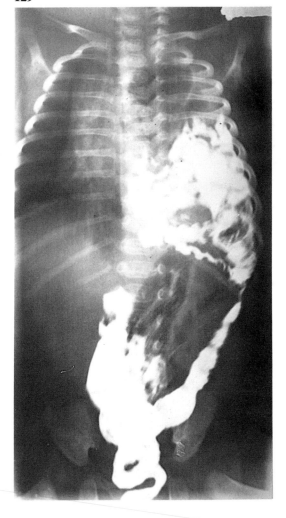

128 and 129 Diaphragmatic hernia is a neonatal emergency which usually results from herniation of the bowel into the thorax through a defect in the left hemidiaphragm. Most cases present with severe respiratory distress in the first hour of life resulting from the infant swallowing air which inflates the stomach and small bowel causing collapse of the left lung and displacement of the mediastinum to the right. In severe cases the stomach, small bowel and left lobe of the liver may lie in the left hemithorax during fetal life resulting in hypoplasia of the lungs and consequently a more adverse prognosis. **129** shows the same infant as seen in **128** in whom a barium meal has been performed. Loops of bowel with contrast medium are seen in the left hemithorax.

130

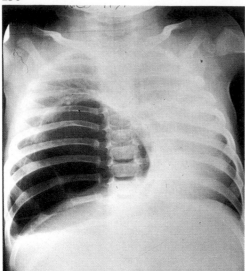

131

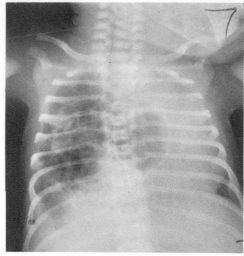

130 Pneumatocoele. A pneumatocoele occurs most commonly as a complication of staphylococcal pneumonia. It may rupture into the pleura causing a tension pneumothorax and acute onset of dyspnoea.

131 Congenital lung cyst. In this figure a large cyst in the right hemithorax can be seen. There may be no abnormal clinical signs but more commonly the anomaly causes a problem due to infection or expansion as the result of a ball valve tension cyst developing. In this case the infant presented with respiratory distress at the age of 1 month and treatment was by surgical removal of the cyst.

132

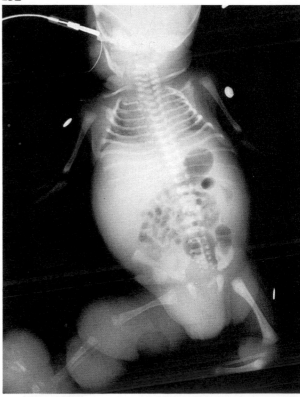

132 Arterio-venous fistula is a rare but treatable cause of severe heart failure in the newborn. The fistula may occur anywhere, but intracranial ones are commonest. In this case the infant had a fistula of the right leg resulting in gross swelling which is obvious on the radiograph. Also seen are enlargement of the heart and liver due to congestive cardiac failure.

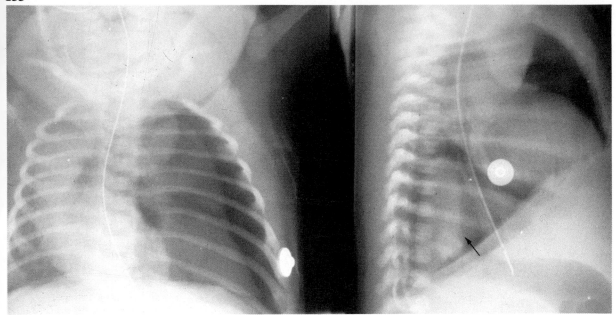

133 Pulmonary sequestration is said to occur when a lobe of the lung, usually the left lower lobe, develops but has no connection with the tracheo-bronchial tree or pulmonary blood supply. Resection of the sequestered lobe is necessary as it is prone to repeated infections. In this infant the sequestered lobe is outlined well because of the concomitant presence of a left pneumothorax (arrow).

134

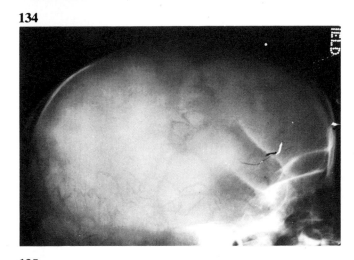

135

134 and 135 Cleidocranial dysostosis. The classical radiological feature of cleidocranial dysostosis is absence of the clavicles which can be seen in this chest radiograph. Clinically the condition is suspected because the patient is able to approximate the shoulder to the sternum and the diagnosis is confirmed by palpation. The condition causes no long-term problems for the individual but cephalopelvic disproportion may result in obstetric problems for the fetus. **134** shows the lateral skull radiograph of an infant with cleidocranial dysostosis. The skull is very soft with wide fontanelles and sutures. The condition is inherited as an autosomal dominant.

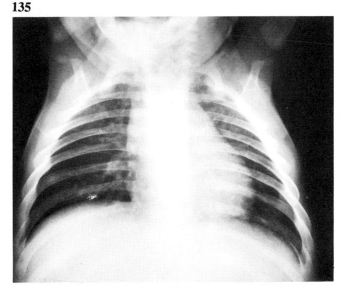

136 Anomalous pulmonary venous drainage. In anomalous pulmonary venous drainage the pulmonary veins drain into the right atrium. Survival is impossible unless there is a communication between the left and right sides of the heart. The infant presents with gross cyanosis and a chest radiograph shows a normal cardiac outline and plethoric lung fields. Later right atrial and ventricular hypertrophy occur as seen in this figure and the abnormal pulmonary venous drainage can be seen on the right (arrow).

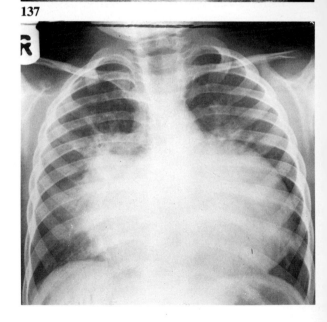

137 Endomyocardial fibroelastosis. This may present at any time within the first 6 months of life. Clinically the infant shows non-specific malaise or cardiac failure. A chest radiograph reveals gross enlargement of the heart and an ECG may show signs of heart block. Response to anti-failure therapy is usually good to begin with but the long-term prognosis is often poor.

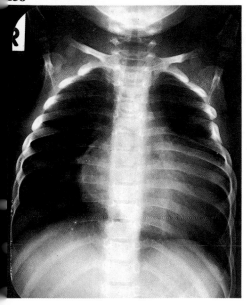

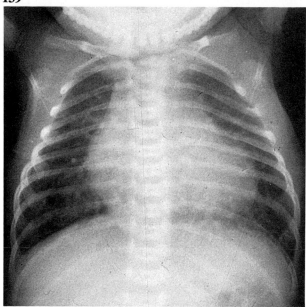

138 Anomalous left coronary artery.
In this condition the left coronary artery originates in the pulmonary artery and not from the aorta. Consequently there is myocardial ischaemia and heart failure. This radiograph shows enlargement of the left ventricle. Clinically the infant is not cyanosed and does not have a cardiac murmur.

139 Pulmonary oedema may result from fluid overload or any condition that causes left ventricular failure. Note the uniform cardiomegaly and pulmonary plethora. Clinically the infant is likely to show signs of respiratory distress and may be cyanosed. Auscultation of the chest may reveal uniform crepitations.

140

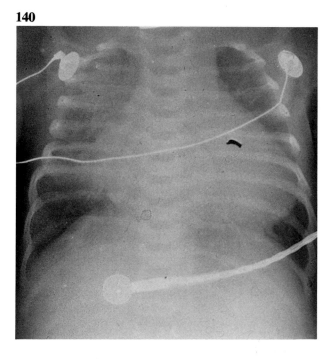

140 Coarctation of the aorta is usually preductal when presenting clinically in the neonatal period. Persistence of a right to left shunt through the duct results in palpable femoral pulses and clinical presentation may be that of cardiac failure alone. This radiograph shows marked cardiomegaly and pulmonary oedema. The diagnosis of preductal coarctation may be suspected if there are asymmetric pulses in the right and left arms.

141 Transposition of the great vessels. Transposition is one of the commoner congenital cardiac anomalies presenting in the neonatal period. In classical transposition the pulmonary trunk arises from the left ventricle and the aorta from the right ventricle. Postnatal survival depends upon the persistence of fetal communication between the lesser and greater circulations and a classical clinical presentation is of an infant initially thought to be normal who then collapses at about the age of 3 days with severe irreversible cyanosis. Nitrogen washout confirms the cardiac aetiology of the cyanosis. The radiograph reveals a distinctive cardiac shadow resembling an egg on its side. Emergency treatment is required by atrial balloon septostomy.

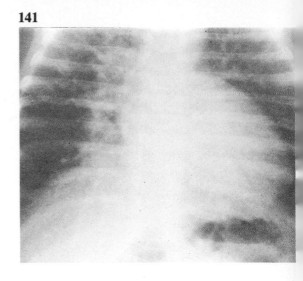

142 Chylothorax is a term used to describe the persistence of chyle, or lymphatic fluid within the thorax. A chylothorax arising spontaneously is very rare, the commonest cause being ligation of the thoracic duct following cardiac surgery. Chylothorax is usually seen on the left as in this case.

142

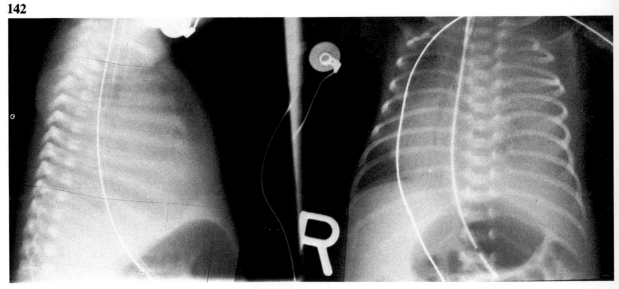

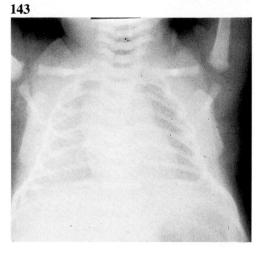

143 Neuropathic chest. In this radiograph the noteworthy feature is the bell-shaped thorax in which the ribs are abnormally short and horizontal. Such a thorax may be seen in a variety of conditions in which there is prenatal weakness of the thoracic muscles due usually to a neurological abnormality. In such patients the presentation is most commonly of respiratory distress with marked diaphragmatic respiration. Patients with Lejeunc's asphyxiating thoracic dystrophy have such a chest, short arms and may have polydactyly.

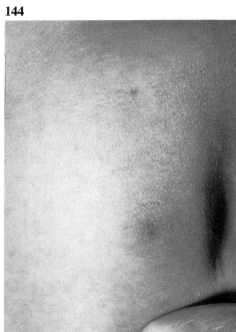

144 Accessory nipple. Accessory nipples may be single or multiple and may occur anywhere on the thorax or abdomen between the mid-axillary line and the mid-line. They have no ominous significance but may require removal for cosmetic reasons.

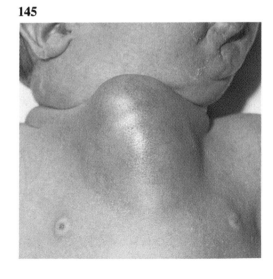

145 Teratoma. A teratoma may occur at any site in the newborn infant. This figure shows an anterior mediastinal teratoma which was associated with respiratory distress. A teratoma may occur anywhere in the mediastinum and the first indication may arise from a chest radiograph. Treatment is surgical.

5 The abdomen

Abdominal distension is most commonly a sign of intestinal obstruction in the newborn, although the following figures show other causes as well.

146

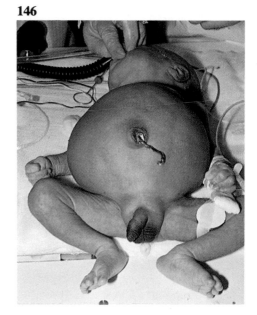

146 Abdominal distension: ileal atresia. This figure shows an infant with ileal atresia who did not present for treatment until the age of 3 days. Note how gross abdominal distension can become at this age.

147

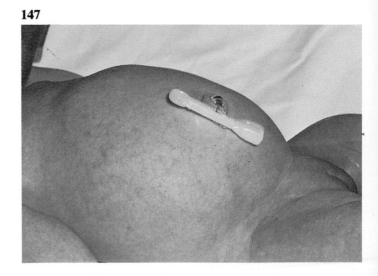

147 Abdominal distension: septicaemia. Abdominal distension is commonly seen in neonatal septicaemia and improves spontaneously as the infection is treated. It is probably due to ileus of the small and large bowel.

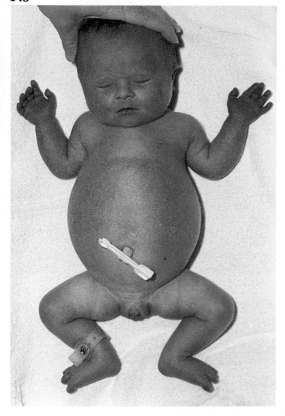

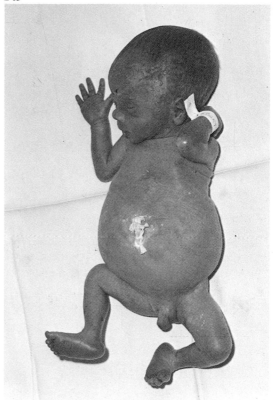

148 Abdominal distension: ascites. Ascites may complicate any neonatal condition in which there is fluid overload but is most commonly due to prenatal congestive cardiac failure due to haemolytic disease (see **20** and **21**). Prenatal haemolysis is most commonly due to rhesus incompatibility. Note that this baby also has Down's syndrome (see **269** to **275**).

149 Abdominal distension: masses. Unexplained large masses in the neonatal abdomen are usually renal. This baby has bilateral hydronephrosis in association with absence of the abdominal musculature, a condition known as the "prune belly syndrome".

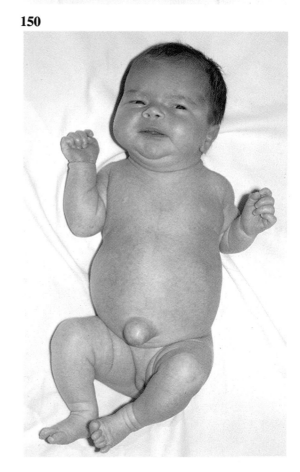

150 Abdominal distension: umbilical hernia. This figure shows a baby in whom ascites is complicated by a large umbilical hernia.

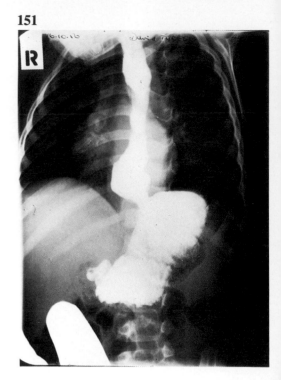

151 Hiatus hernia usually presents with effortless, non-bile stained vomiting which may on occasion be complicated by aspiration pneumonia. In later infancy the patient may present as failure to thrive with an iron deficiency anaemia. This figure shows oesophageal dilatation and gastric reflux during a barium swallow investigation.

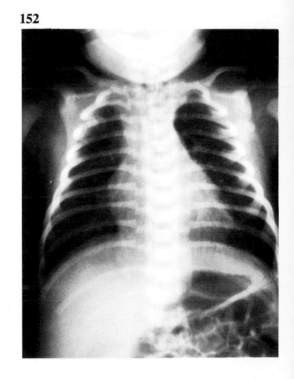

152 and 153 Oesophageal atresia occurs commonly associated with a tracheo-oesophageal fistula. The presenting signs in the newborn period are most commonly due to the atresia which results in inability to swallow and spilling of both saliva and milk into the trachea. The infant presents characteristically with a choking attack in the early hours of life which is relieved by suction. The initial investigation involves attempting to pass a tube into the stomach. **152** and **153** show failure of the naso-gastric tube to pass the upper thorax. Note how a diagnosis of tracheo-oesophageal fistula may also be made from these radiographs since there is air in the stomach and small intestine and in the oesophagus (**153**) which could only have got there via the trachea. On occasion the doctor or nurse may be misled by a naso-gastric tube curling up in the blind upper oesophageal pouch or as a result of the tube passing down the trachea. It is advisable to confirm that the tip of the tube is in the stomach by auscultating the abdomen while injecting air and by aspirating gastric contents and testing these with litmus.

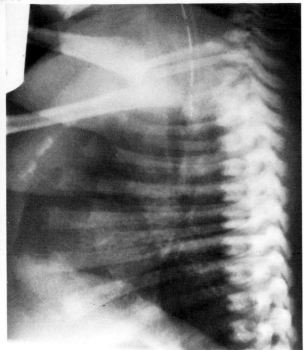

153

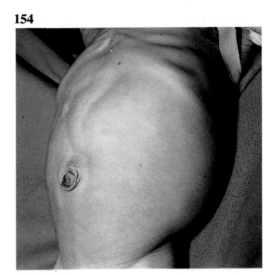

154

154 Pyloric stenosis usually presents at the age of 4 to 8 weeks but may be present at birth. The characteristic symptom is projectile vomiting during and immediately after feeds which is not bile-stained. There is also constipation. The infant fails to thrive. Inspection of the abdomen during a feed may reveal waves of peristalsis in the epigastrium as seen in this figure. Palpation, from the left-hand side, may reveal the hypertrophic pyloric muscle as a mass about the size of an olive against the right lateral aspect of the first lumbar vertebra. Treatment is usually surgical, but some physicians persist with antispasmodic therapy.

155 Perforated duodenal ulcer. Duodenal ulcer in the newborn is rare. It may cause either catastrophic gastrointestinal haemorrhage or pneumoperitoneum following perforation.

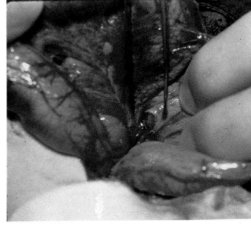

155

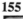

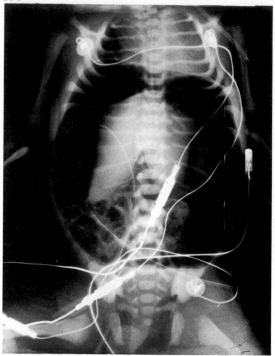

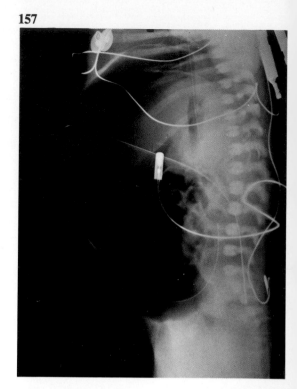

156 and 157 Pneumoperitoneum. This figure shows gross abdominal gaseous distension due to perforation. The infant presents in a state of shock. Perforation in this case was due to rupture of the stomach which occurred as a complication of intubation of the oesophagus and incorrect assisted ventilation. **157** is a lateral radiograph of the infant shown in **156**.

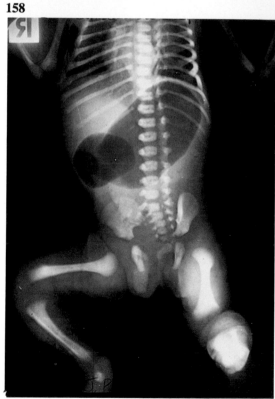

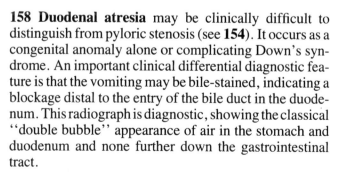

158 Duodenal atresia may be clinically difficult to distinguish from pyloric stenosis (see **154**). It occurs as a congenital anomaly alone or complicating Down's syndrome. An important clinical differential diagnostic feature is that the vomiting may be bile-stained, indicating a blockage distal to the entry of the bile duct in the duodenum. This radiograph is diagnostic, showing the classical "double bubble" appearance of air in the stomach and duodenum and none further down the gastrointestinal tract.

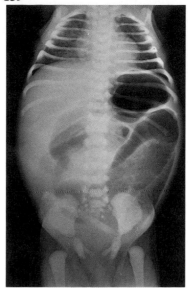

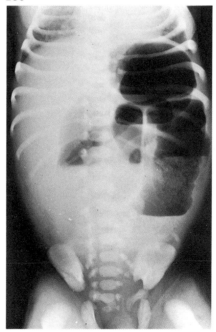
160

159 and 160 Small intestinal atresia. This most commonly involves the ileum, though it may occur anywhere in the small bowel and in more than one place in the same infant. The clinical features are those of bowel obstruction usually becoming apparent on the second day of life. This radiograph shows dilated small bowel with fluid levels in the erect film (**160**) but no gas in the large bowel.

161 Obstructive jaundice is suspected clinically by its yellow-green hue in contrast to the more common neonatal jaundice which is orange-red. Obstructive jaundice becomes apparent during the second week of life and is most commonly due to either neonatal hepatitis or atresia of the bile ducts but may be seen as a complication of parenteral nutrition. Depending on the aetiology, the jaundice may resolve spontaneously after several weeks or be permanent if surgical treatment is not undertaken. Note in this case that the infant shows also abdominal distension and marked ascites. The baby had atresia of the bile ducts which was treated by anastomosis of the porta hepatis and jejunum.

161

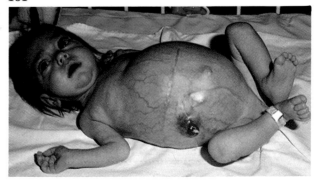

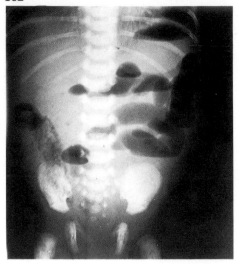

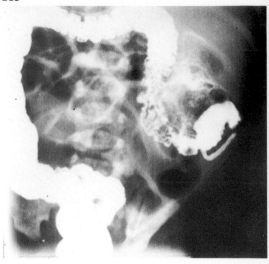

162 and 163 Milk inspissation may occur as a form of intestinal obstruction seen in infants fed with formula. A variety of explanations has been offered including over-feeding but the cause is most probably due to formula containing too much long chain saturated fatty acids which form insoluble soaps resulting in indigestible milk curd. Realization of this problem has led to most modern formulas being made with appropriate fat mixtures that result in normal digestion and absorption. The radiograph shows numerous fluid levels throughout the small bowel and is similar to the film seen in meconium ileus. The milk curds causing intestinal blockage can be seen in the right iliac fossa. **163** is of a gastrograffin enema showing narrowing of the large bowel in the ileo-caecal region. The enema may have a curative as well as a diagnostic role.

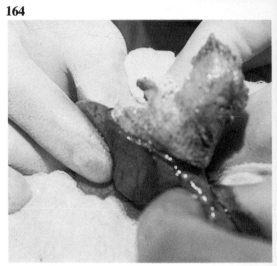

164 Milk inspissation. This figure shows milk curd being removed from the small bowel at operation.

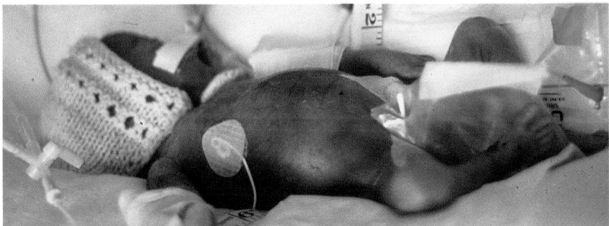

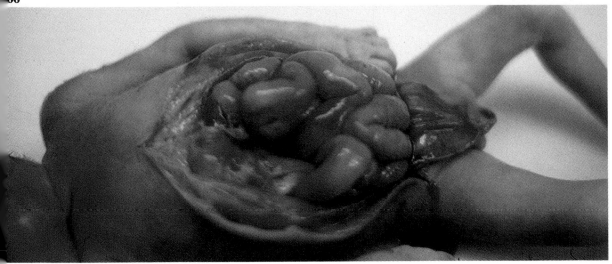

165 and 166 Necrotizing enterocolitis (NEC) occurs most commonly in pre-term infants and those who are ill for other reasons. The early clinical signs include abdominal distension and the presence of blood in the stools which may initially be microscopic. If the disease progresses, vomiting and ileus occur. This pre-term infant shows an advanced stage of NEC in which there is distension of the abdomen and haemorrhage into the abdominal wall. **166** is of a postmortem examination and shows the characteristically grossly distended ischaemic and haemorrhagic appearance of the bowel.

167

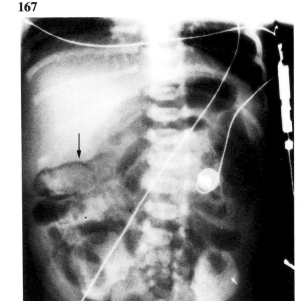

168

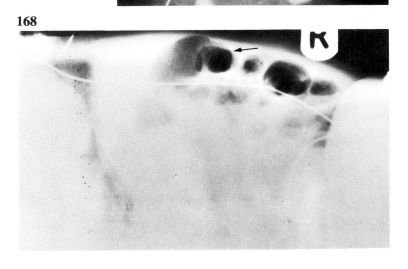

167 and 168 Necrotizing enterocolitis: radiology. There are a number of radiological features which help in the diagnosis of NEC. An early sign is a foamy appearance of the bowel content. The classical sign is pneumatosis intestinalis – air in the wall of the bowel or stomach. A late sign is pneumoperitoneum or air in the hepatic ducts. **167** shows the foamy appearance of the bowel contents and pneumatosis intestinalis (arrow). A lateral radiograph (**168**) also shows clear evidence of pneumatosis intestinalis (arrow).

169

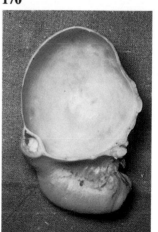

169 Choledochal cyst. Cystic dilatation of the bile duct due to obstruction results in a choledochal cyst. The size of the cyst may vary and symptoms in the neonatal period are rare. A choledochal cyst presenting in the newborn is usually large. The infant has a right-sided abdominal mass and is jaundiced. This radiograph shows a fluid-filled mass in the right side of the abdomen.

170

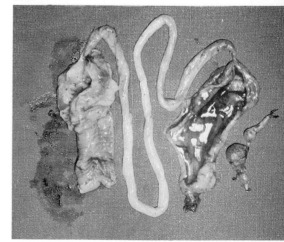

171

170 and 171 Duplication cyst arises from malformation of the viscera resulting in a cyst which is most commonly found in the abdomen but which may occasionally be intrathoracic. They are generally attached to the bowel and have a similar epithelial structure. They may be of any size: larger ones are often palpable. The operation specimen shown in **171** shows a tubular duplication cyst which has been dissected out together with a small portion of normal bowel to which it is attached.

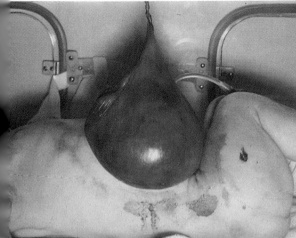

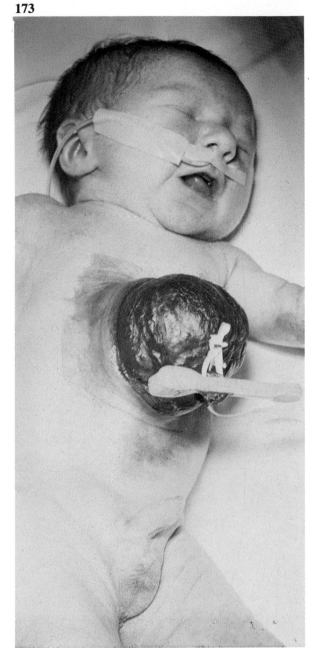

172 and 173 Exomphalos is caused by failure of the gut to return to the abdominal cavity in early fetal life (10 weeks). There is an associated muscular defect of the anterior abdominal wall. In **172** the intestines are covered by a membranous sac which is suspended from the umbilical cord. In exomphalos the membranous sac may often rupture (**174**). In the case illustrated in **173** the patient presented somewhat later and the membranous covering to the bowel has dried.

174

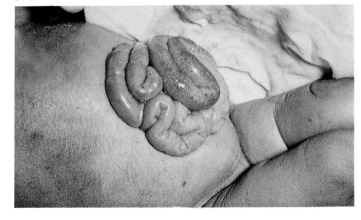

174 Gastroschisis. This baby has an exomphalos which has ruptured leading to spillage of the intestines on the anterior abdominal surface. The condition is more serious due to desiccation of the gut wall and necrosis.

175 and 176 Volvulus occurs due to a mesenteric abnormality which results in the bowel being unattached to the posterior abdominal wall except at the duodenum and proximal colon. Consequently the small intestine may twist on itself resulting in obstruction and possible gangrene. The radiological appearances are variable but usually show some gas in the duodenum and a hazy appearance of the rest of the abdomen as seen in **175**. In **176** a radiograph taken in the erect position shows fluid levels in addition to the features shown in **175**.

175

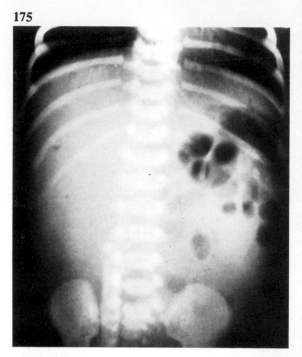

176

177

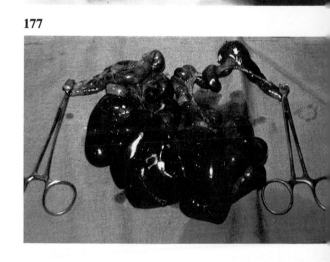

177 Gangrenous bowel. This operation specimen shows gangrenous dilated bowel removed at operation. Gangrene of the bowel may result from a number of conditions including necrotizing enterocolitis and volvulus.

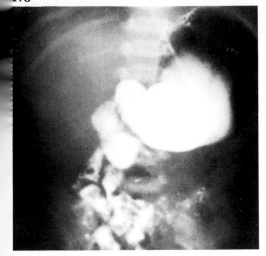

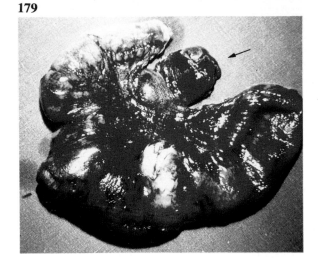

178 Malrotation of the intestine. Malrotation may be asymptomatic or present with intestinal obstruction due to volvulus or compression of the small bowel by the caecum. This figure shows a barium meal and follow-through radiograph in which the caecum is misplaced in the right upper quadrant of the abdomen and displaces the small intestine.

179 Meckel's diverticulum occurs when there is failure of the proximal part of the mesenteric duct to obliterate. The diverticulum usually arises from the ileum. Meckel's diverticulum is commonly asymptomatic but symptoms can arise from haemorrhage or perforation due to erosion of ectopic gastric mucosa in the diverticulum. This figure shows an operative specimen in which the terminal ileum and caecum have been removed together with a Meckel's diverticulum (arrow).

180

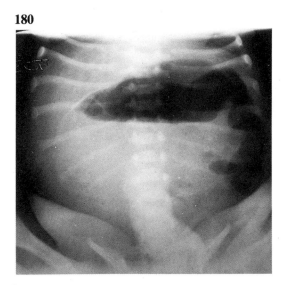

181

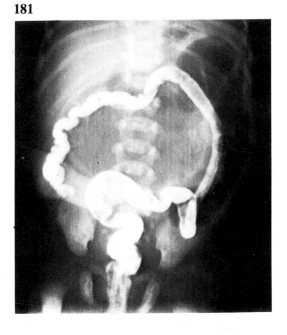

180 and 181 Meconium peritonitis often arises *in utero* resulting in a newborn baby who presents with abdominal distension, respiratory distress and oedema of the anterior abdominal wall. If perforation of the bowel occurs after delivery the signs of peritonitis follow rapidly. The classical association of meconium peritonitis is with either meconium ileus in cystic fibrosis or bowel atresia, but often no cause is found. **180** shows an abdominal radiograph in which there is diffuse calcification in the peritoneum, a classical radiological sign of this condition. **181** demonstrates a gastrograffin enema performed in the patient illustrated in **180**. The enema demonstrates patency of the large intestine and the presence of a micro-colon.

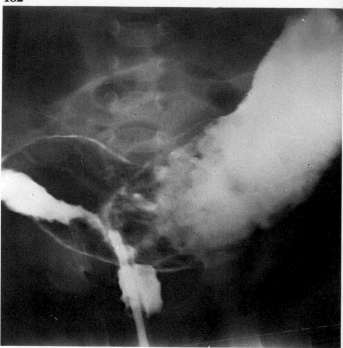

182 Hirschprung's disease is due to aganglionosis of a segment of the colon and may present during the first week of life with delayed passage of meconium coupled with abdominal distension. Although constipation is the rule, some patients may present with overflow diarrhoea. In this radiograph the barium enema shows gross dilatation of the large bowel proximal to the short aganglionic segment.

183

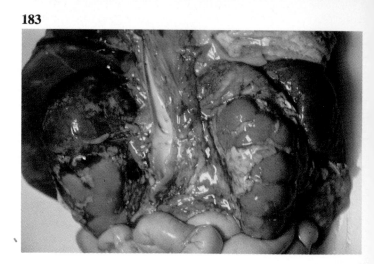

183 Adrenal haemorrhage may occur in the newborn secondary to trauma. A small adrenal haemorrhage may be asymptomatic but a large one can be followed by hypovolaemia and circulatory collapse. Secondary adrenal insufficiency may result but this is seldom total.

184

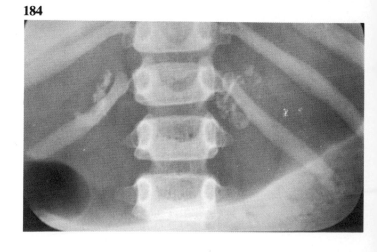

184 Adrenal calcification. This occurs a few weeks after adrenal haemorrhage and may remain as a permanent radiological curiosity. This radiograph shows bilateral adrenal calcification.

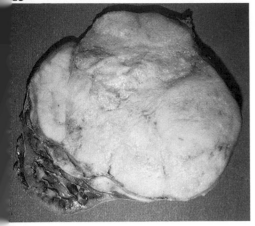

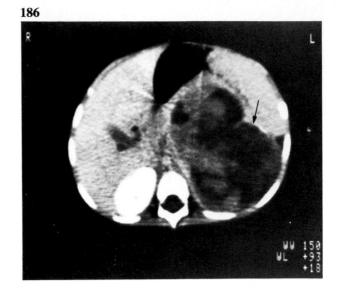

185 and 186 Wilm's tumour (nephro-blastoma). This is the commonest solid tumour in childhood and may occasionally be present at birth. The clinical sign is of an intra-abdominal mass which may be massive as seen in the operative specimen in **185**. **186** is of a CAT scan showing a large retroperitoneal mass which is partly cystic lying where the left kidney would be expected (arrows). This was a nephroblastoma.

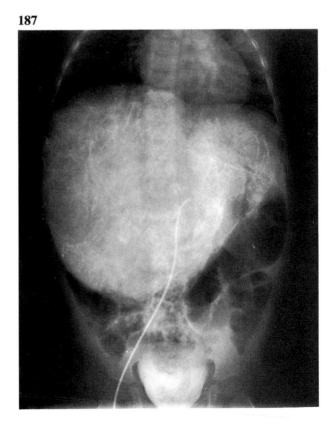

187 Hepatoblastoma is a rare tumour that may present as an abdominal mass in the neonatal period. A plain abdominal radiograph may show a large space-occupying mass in the region of the liver which may be calcified. This figure shows an angiogram performed via the umbilical vein demonstrating involvement of both the right and left lobe of the liver.

188

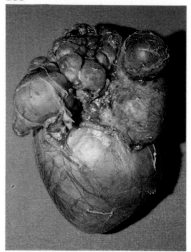

189

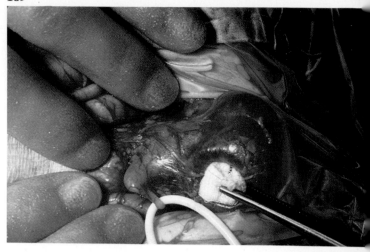

188 Multicystic kidney. Multi-cystic kidneys may be palpated in the newborn as a mass in the loin. There is very little or no functioning renal tissue, the kidney consisting of a series of multiloculated cysts. Treatment is by excision. In many cases the other kidney is also abnormal.

189 and 190 Hydronephrosis in the newborn occurs most commonly due to obstruction at the bladder neck or at the pelvo-ureteric junction. In **189** gross enlargement of the kidney can be easily seen and the pelvo-ureteric junction is illustrated by the white catheter behind the non-obstructed ureter distal to the obstruction. **190** shows on the left part of a plain abdomen X-ray in which the left kidney is seen through a stomach that has been blown up with air. Note the dilated calyces (arrows). On the right a similar view is seen; only the calyces have now been outlined with dye injected via a ureterostomy.

190

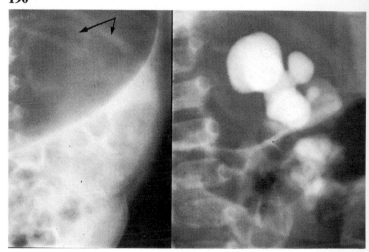

191

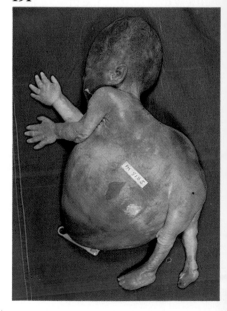

191 Urethral atresia. This stillborn baby was found to have atresia of the urethra at necropsy resulting in gross distension of the bladder, ureters and kidneys. The bladder contained 400 ml of urine.

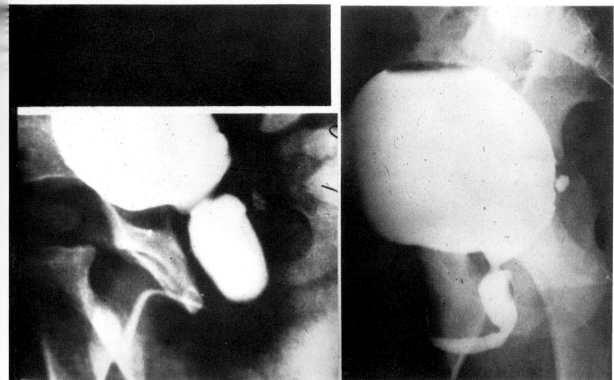

192 Urinary obstruction. Failure to pass urine may be due to a number of reasons at the vesico-urethral area, two of which are illustrated in this figure. The radiograph on the left shows a micturating cysto-urethrogram in a patient with urethral valves. Note the grossly dilated proximal urethra and very narrow urinary stream distal to the valve. Urethral valves occur only in boys and are treated by cautery. On the right is a cysto-urethrogram of a neuropathic bladder in an infant with myelomeningocoele. Note the relatively normal outflow tract despite the gross enlargement of the bladder.

193

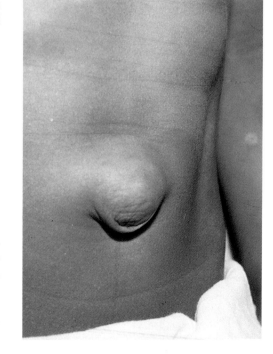

193 Umbilical hernia arises due to separation of the rectus muscles with herniation of the omentum and on some occasions bowel. The hernia is skin-covered, the size varies considerably, but since these hernias are wide-necked, intestinal obstruction does not occur. Umbilical hernias disappear spontaneously as the rectus muscles become stronger and most are gone by the age of 2 years.

194 Single umbilical artery. The umbilical cord normally contains three vessels: two arteries and one vein. Occasionally one of the arteries is absent. Usually this is an isolated, minor congenital anomaly but it should alert the clinician to search for other abnormalities since a single umbilical artery may be associated with multiple congenital anomalies, in particular congenital renal anomalies.

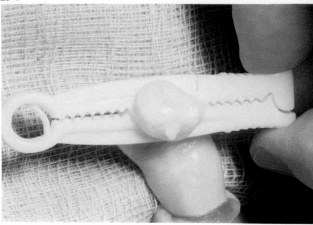

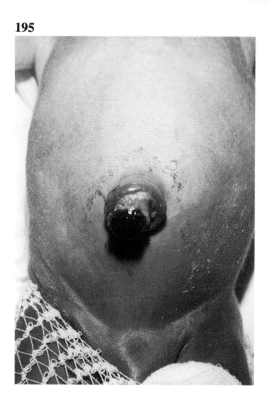

195 Patent vitelline (omphalo-mesenteric) duct. During early fetal life the vitelline duct connects the yolk sac to the primitive bowel. The vitelline duct normally obliterates and atrophies in the course of fetal development, but on occasion may persist and presents shortly after birth as a channel through which intestinal contents pass from the umbilicus. In this figure, bowel has prolapsed through the patent vitelline duct. Treatment is by excision.

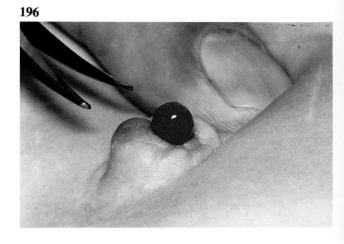

196 Umbilical polyp. An umbilical polyp may arise when the vitelline duct fails to obliterate and atrophy completely. The duct persists as a blind channel passing from the umbilicus into the abdomen and is recognized as a red nodule at the umbilicus. Treatment is by excision taking care to exclude a patent connection to the bowel.

197

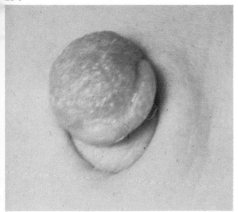

197 Umbilical granuloma results from an overgrowth of granulation tissue at the umbilicus. It is prone to irritation and may bleed. Treatment is by cautery.

198 Hepatosplenomegaly. Hepatic enlargement may be found in normal neonates but hepatosplenomegaly as seen in this figure is always pathological. There are many causes of hepatosplenomegaly including prenatal infection (see **308**) and haemolytic anaemia (see **20**). The discovery of hepatosplenomegaly calls for urgent further investigation.

198

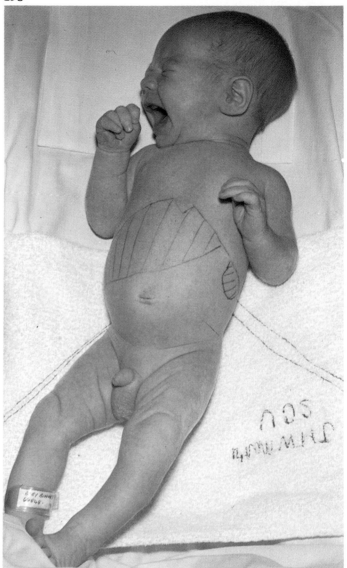

199

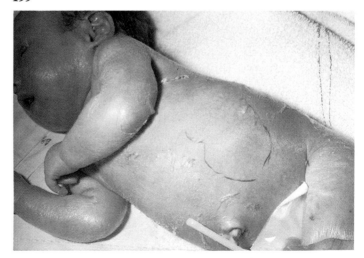

199 Splenomegaly may occur as an isolated clinical finding. The most common cause is haemolytic anaemia, but prenatal or neonatal infection should be considered. Portal thrombosis is a rare cause.

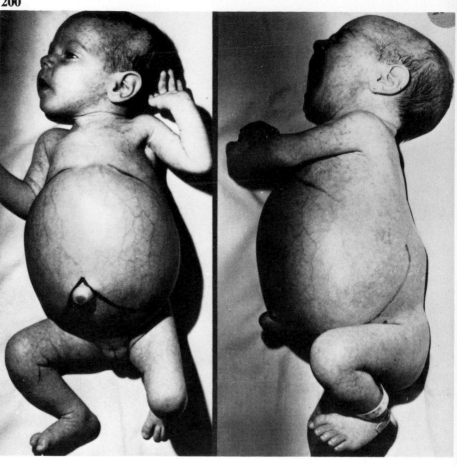

201

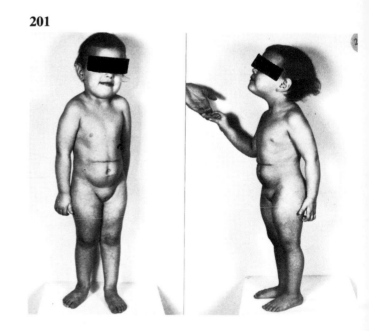

200 and 201 Neuroblastoma may
present in the neonatal period usually as
an abdominal mass. The tumour arises
either from the adrenal gland or the
para-aortic sympathetic ganglia.
Metastases are often widespread at the
time of presentation. The prognosis is
variable and better in those cases presenting under 1 year of age. The infant
shown in **200** had a huge upper abdominal mass which was due to a neuroblastoma but which could not be distinguished clinically from a hepatoblastoma (see **187**) or a Wilm's tumour
(see **185**). **201** shows the same patient as
that depicted in **200** at the age of 3 years
when she was clinically well.

6 The pelvis and perineum

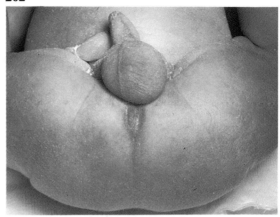

202

203

202 and 203 Imperforate anus is recognized either by inspection of the natal cleft or by failure of an apparently normal newborn to pass meconium. Cases are divided into "high" and "low" depending on whether the atresia is above or below the supralevator muscle. The majority of high anal atresias have a fistulous communication with the bladder in boys or the genital tract in girls leading to passage of meconium per urethram or per vaginam and a possible delay in establishing diagnosis. In a low anal atresia there may be a fistula to the natal cleft. The classical method of making the diagnosis is to perform a radiograph of the infant with a radiopaque object strapped to the external anal orifice. As seen in **203** there is failure of gas to fill the anal rectum and anal canal, illustrating a high anal atresia.

204

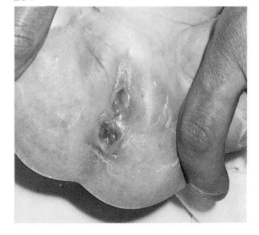

204 Imperforate anus and rectovaginal fistula.
This figure shows clearly the fistula which may occur between a high imperforate anus and the posterior vaginal wall.

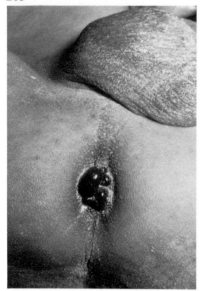

205 Rectal prolapse may be seen at birth in association with anomalies such as exstrophy of the bladder or any other condition causing raised intra-abdominal pressure. The prolapse usually remits spontaneously but may need manual replacement.

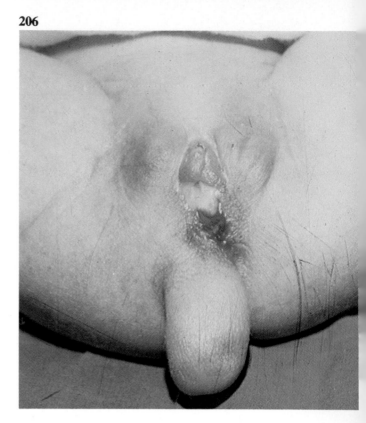

206 Perineal lipoma is recognized immediately following birth on inspection of the infant. The tumours occur most often in the lumbosacral area and may overlie a spina bifida occulta or an abnormality of the cauda equina. They may be associated with a lower motor neurone lesion of the legs and a neuropathic bladder.

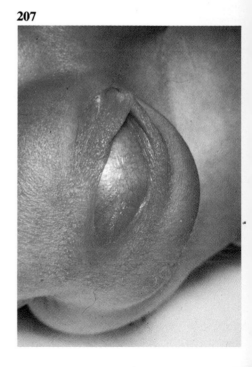

207 Hydrocolpos results from retention of uterine and vaginal secretions by an imperforate hymen. In this figure the mass presenting at the introitus is due to a hydrocolpos and incision of the hymen cures the swelling. Hydrocolpos may present as a lower abdominal swelling. In such cases it is essential to examine the perineum when the diagnosis of hydrocolpos may save the patient from a laparotomy.

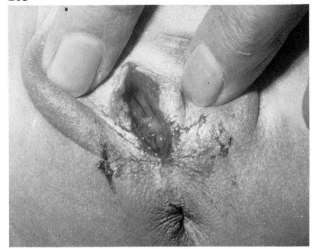

208 Pseudomenstruation. Vaginal bleeding is not uncommon in the first week of life. The cause is withdrawal from the high oestrogen level to which the baby has been exposed *in utero*. Vaginal bleeding is self-limiting and the mother may be reassured with confidence.

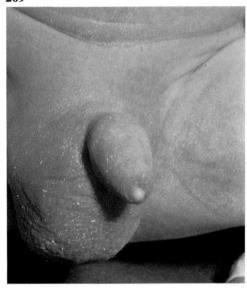

209 Epstein's pearls are small, sebaceous cysts most commonly seen on the penis or scrotum but which may also be seen on the palate. They burst spontaneously and do not recur.

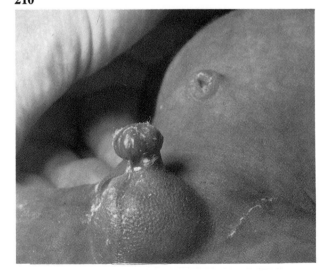

210 Hypospadias results from failure of normal development of the urethra. This figure illustrates a glandular hypospadias in which the urethra terminates on the ventral surface of the penis proximal to the glans. The prepuce has failed to fuse resulting in a hooded prepuce and the angulation of the penile shaft is known as chordee. Circumcision is contraindicated as the foreskin is needed in the repair of the hypospadias.

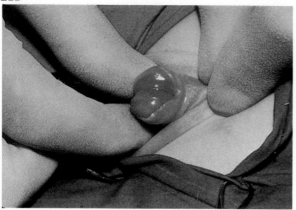

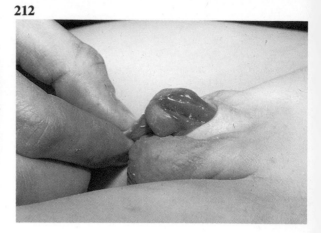

211 and 212 Epispadias. In epispadias the urethral opening is on the dorsal aspect of the glans penis. The opening may be small or, as in the case shown in **211**, large enough to form a furrow bisecting the glans. A further case of epispadias illustrating failure of development of the dorsal aspect of the prepuce is shown in **212**.

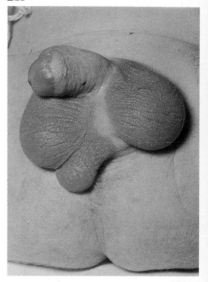

213 Trifid scrotum is a rare variant of the commoner bifid scrotum in which the scrotum is divided into two halves each containing a testis. Bifid or trifid scrotum is important because of the association of other perineal abnormalities: in this case there was hypospadias and an imperforate anus.

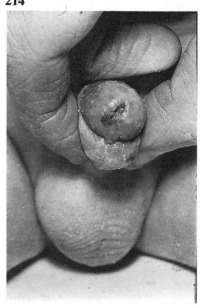

214 Meatal ulcer is normally seen only in circumcised boys. It consists of a superficial ulcer surrounding the urethral meatus which results from ammoniacal dermatitis. The majority heal spontaneously but occasionally meatal stenosis may result.

215 Exstrophy of the bladder. This rare condition results from failure of development of the lower half of the anterior abdominal wall including deep structures such as the symphysis pubis and anterior bladder wall. In this figure the exstrophy involves the bladder and vagina. The labia are widely split and the anus can be seen below.

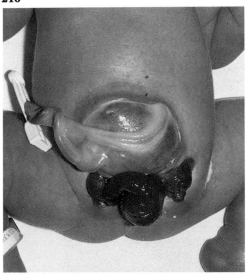

216 Vesico-intestinal fissure results from abnormal development of the lower half of the abdominal wall. Features of vesico-intestinal fissure seen in this patient include exomphalos, bladder exstrophy and a blind colon which is associated with ano-rectal agenesis. Vesico-intestinal fissure is also referred to as ectopia cloacae.

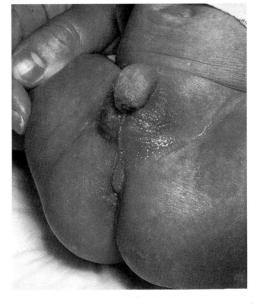

217 Adrenogenital syndrome. The adrenogenital syndrome results from an enzymic block of glucocorticoid biosynthesis resulting in excess secretion of androgens and masculinization of the female fetus. The baby may be born superficially resembling a male with fusion of the labia majora to look like a scrotum and clitoral hypertrophy that resembles a penis. Diagnostic clues arise from absence of the testes and apparent hypospadias.

218 Ambiguous genitalia. Inspection of the external genitalia in this patient shows that the scrotum is bifid and contains gonads. The clinician should beware of assuming that the gonads are testes in patients where the external genitalia are not totally normal. The gonad may contain ovarian tissue resulting in an ovo-testis or there may be an ovary on one side and a testis on the other. The clinical examination of patients with ambiguous genitalia should include a rectal examination to palpate for a cervix and careful examination of the external inguinal orifices for undescended gonads. Investigations include a "cloacogram" in which dye injected into the urethra may pass not only into the bladder but also in the vagina and may or may not illustrate a cervix. Karyotyping is essential and laparoscopy may be indicated to see the internal genitalia. In rare cases gonadal biopsy may be indicated both for histological examination and further chromosome analysis.

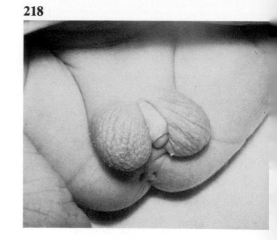

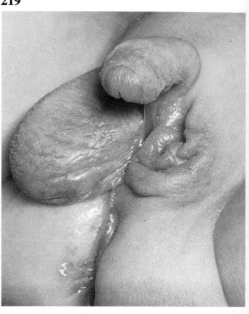

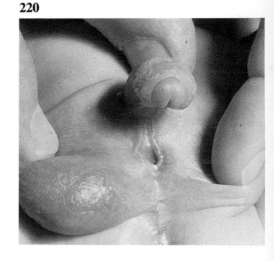

219 and 220 Hermaphrodite. In this patient there was fusion of the labio-scrotal folds with a gonad on the right and a perineal hypospadias. Investigation of this patient revealed that the urethral opening led to both the vagina and bladder. The scrotal gonad was a testis but on the left hand side the internal genitalia were a hemi-uterus, fallopian tube and ovary. Treatment involved removal of the testis, reconstruction of the external genitalia and the patient has subsequently grown up to become a clinically normal female who required further surgery for vaginal reconstruction at puberty.

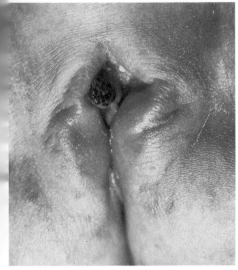

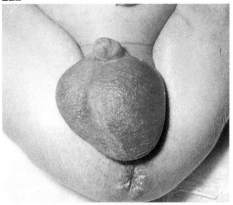

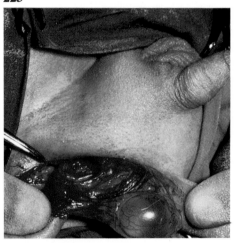

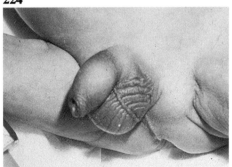

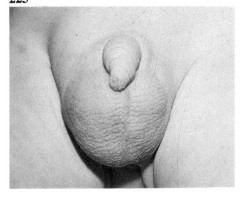

221 Clitoral haemangioma. The clitoris is an unusual site to find a haemangioma.

222 and 223 Hydrocoele. Hydrocoeles arise from an accumulation of fluid in the processus vaginalis which has failed to invaginate following descent of the testis. Hydrocoeles are recognized clinically by being a scrotal mass which transilluminates. **223** shows a hydrocoele at operation where the mass appears as a balloon filled with amber-coloured fluid.

224 Ectopic testis. The testis migrates from the abdominal cavity to the scrotum during the last trimester of pregnancy. Occasionally the testis fails to descend normally or may end in an abnormal site. In this illustration the testis lies in the perineum.

225 Inguinal hernia may occur in the neonatal period when the hernia is usually indirect. It is important that operative repair should be undertaken as soon as possible because there is a high risk of irreducibility and strangulation. Inguinal hernia is rarer in baby girls than baby boys.

7 The back

226

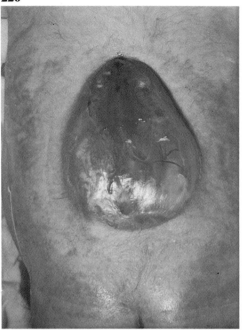

227

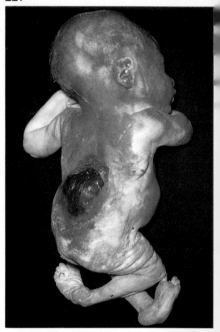

228

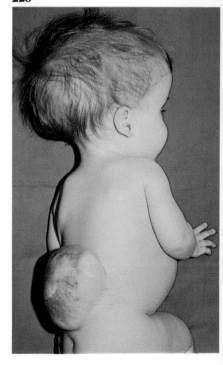

226 Myelomeningocoele results from failure of fusion of the neural tube. This arises most commonly in the lumbo-sacral area but may also occur in the thoraco-lumbar or cervical area. This figure demonstrates exposure of the meninges and the incompletely fused tube. The clinical sequelae of a lumbo-sacral myelo-meningocoele include lower limb paralysis, urinary and faecal incontinence. Hydrocephalus is commonly associated with myelomeningocoele.

227 Myelomeningocoele and raschisis. In this infant with a severe spina bifida the meninges have burst with resultant exposure of underlying neural tissue. Note the severely deformed lower limbs.

228 Myelomeningocoele and hydrocephalus. This infant has a very large head in association with a huge lumbo-sacral myelomeningocoele. This is due to an associated hydrocephalus.

229

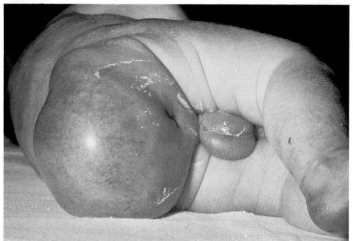

230

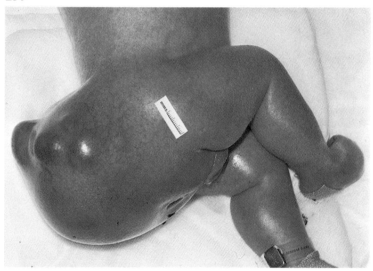

229 and 230 Sacrococcygeal teratoma. These rare tumours present in the first 2 months of life. They consist of a midline sacral swelling that grows caudally and may displace the anus and genitalia. Pelvic extension may occur. Malignant changes can occur in untreated lesions. **230** illustrates the degree to which the tumour may grow in the early neonatal period. Histological examination of the tumour reveals elements of all three germinal layers.

231

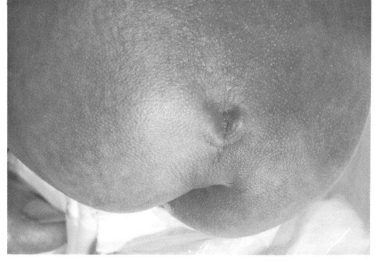

231 Sacrococcygeal pit. A dimple or blind pit in the mid-line of the sacrococcygeal region is not uncommon. Most are benign and require no treatment. When first discovered the pit should be subjected to careful clinical examination to ensure that it is not a sinus extending to the spinal cord.

232 and 233 Scoliosis denotes spinal curvature convex to the right or left. Scoliosis in the newborn is rare but when it occurs is usually associated with a structural anomaly of the vertebral column. Infants with scoliosis are usually female and the condition may be familial. Inspection of the infant in the supine position may lead to equivocal signs, but when the baby is lifted by the armpits (**233**) the scoliosis becomes obvious.

232

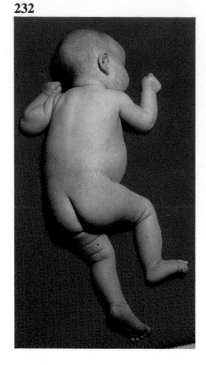

233

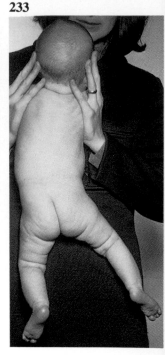

234 Hemivertebra may occur in the cervical or thoracic spine, less commonly in the lumbar spine. An isolated hemivertebra may not be recognized clinically, but can cause abnormal spinal posture and result in scoliosis. More commonly hemivertebrae are multiple as shown in the figure and may be associated with other skeletal abnormalities as in the ribs of this patient.

235 Klippel Feil syndrome is characterized by abnormal fusion of the cervical vertebrae resulting in a short and often wry neck. There may be other associated skeletal defects such as a Sprengel deformity or thoracic hemivertebrae. Involvement of the brachial plexus results in deformities of the hand.

234

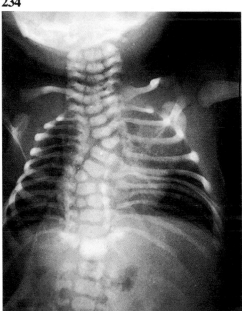

235

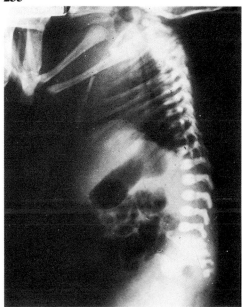

8 The skin

236

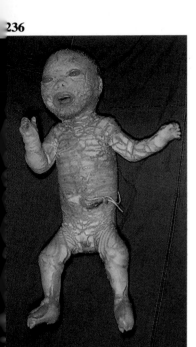

237

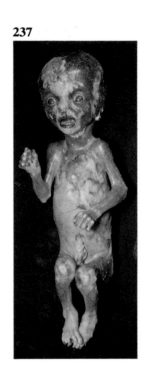

238

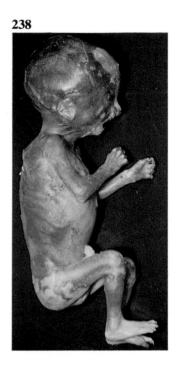

236 Harlequin fetus. A harlequin fetus is the severest form of congenital ichthyosis and is usually fatal. As seen in the figure the skin of the baby is thick, rigid and cracked. The eyes are bright red due to conjunctival oedema, the mouth gapes and other ectodermal structures are hypoplastic. Death results from hypothermia, systemic infection and difficulty in feeding. Inheritance is autosomal recessive.

239

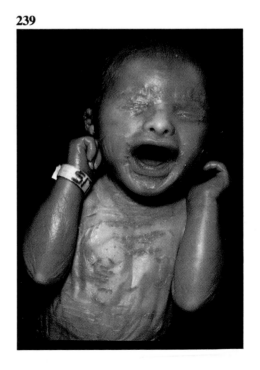

237, 238 and 239 Collodion baby. A collodion baby is a milder form of congenital ichthyosis. As seen in **237** and **238** the infant is born encased in a membrane that is perforated by any hair present on the body. Mobility is limited by the tightness of the membrane until spontaneous peeling begins in the first few days. The underlying skin may be normal or scale to form a new membrane. Clinical management is difficult due to the danger of hypothermia and systemic infection arising from the skin. In the infant shown in **239** a later stage of the condition is illustrated in which peeling has started.

89

240 and 241 Lamellar ichthyosis.
This figure illustrates a further example of congenital ichthyosis which is milder in severity than the preceding illustrations. The scaliness of the skin is widespread and results in both desquamation and pruritus. **241** illustrates the palmar surface of the arm of the baby shown in **240**.

240

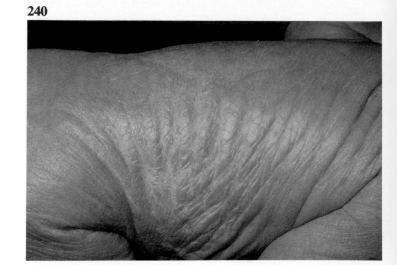

241

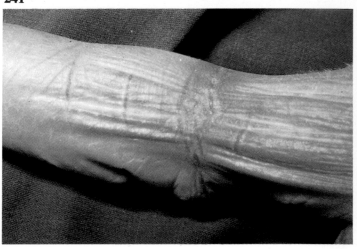

242 and 243 Cavernous haemangioma: minor examples. Cavernous haemangioma is a common finding in the newborn. The baby in **242** has two lesions in the scalp. These are likely to increase in size during the first 6 months of life. The parents should be reassured since spontaneous regression occurs subsequently. **243** is included to illustrate that cavernous haemangiomata may be found anywhere, in this case on the sole of the foot.

242

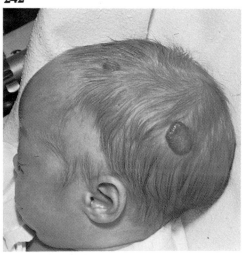

243

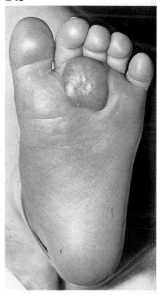

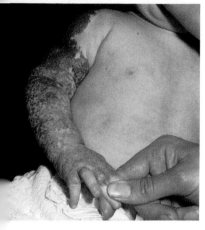

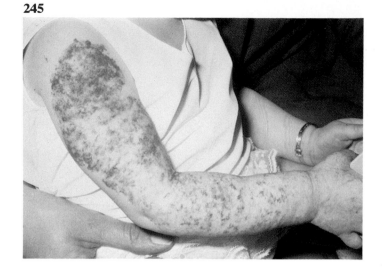

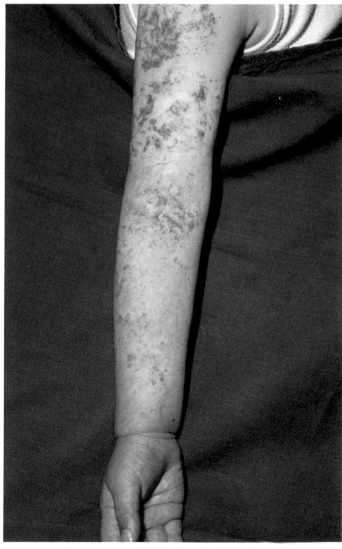

244, 245 and 246 Cavernous haemangioma: a major example. Note the large cavernous haemangioma involving most of the right arm. In **245** it will be noted that by the age of 2 years the lesion shown in **244** has visibly regressed although it is still obvious. By the age of 5 years (**246**) we note that there is further spontaneous resolution of the haemangioma which is now much less unsightly.

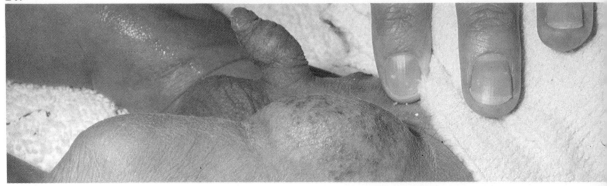

247 Cavernous haemangioma: a major example. On occasion the haemangioma may extend deeply into muscle and form a large blue mass as seen on the anterior aspect of the left thigh in this baby. Very large haemangiomata of this type may be associated with a consumption coagulopathy due to platelet destruction within the haemangioma and systemic haemorrhage may follow.

248

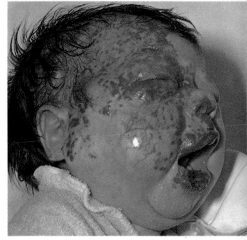

248 Cavernous haemangioma: a major example. This large cavernous haemangioma involving the face interfered with vision. In such rare cases surgical treatment may be necessary.

249

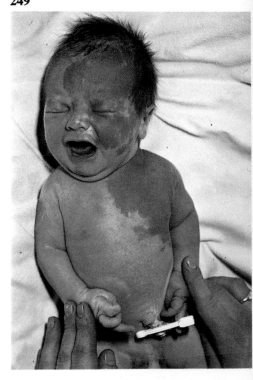

249 and 250 Capillary haemangioma. Capillary haemangioma may be small or very extensive as shown here. No treatment other than cosmetic creams has been available but it is possible that laser beam treatment may prove beneficial in the near future. Capillary haemangiomata do not as a rule fade with age. **250** shows the same infant as illustrated in **249** to demonstrate the extent of the lesion.

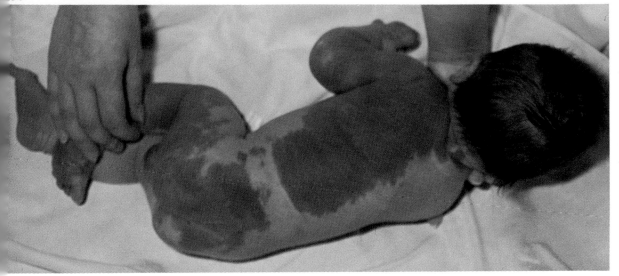

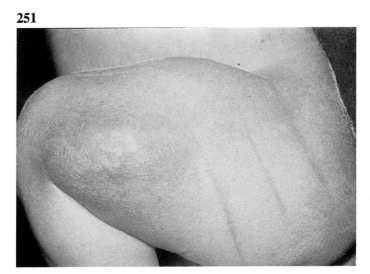

251

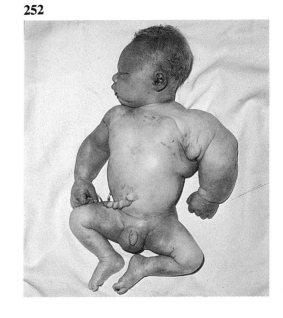

252

251 and 252 Lymphangioma. 251 shows a soft, translucent swelling on the antero-lateral aspect of the left thigh due to accumulation of fluid in lymphatics. The commonest site for a lymphangioma in the newborn is the neck (see **83** cystic hygroma). Lymphangiomata do not resolve spontaneously and treatment by surgery may be complicated. **252** illustrates the deformity which may be associated with a huge lymphangioma involving in this stillborn infant the left arm and hemithorax.

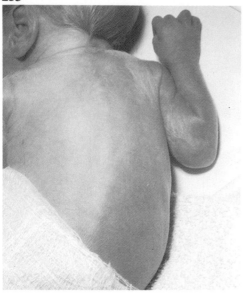

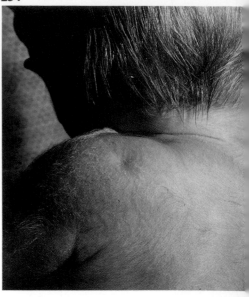

253 Harlequin colour change. This figure shows a newborn infant in whom the right half of the back is vasodilated and the left half pale. The phenomenon although startling is of no pathological significance. If the infant is turned over the harlequin colour change may reverse. Harlequin colour change may last up to a few hours and disappears after the first few months of life. Harlequin colour change is not to be confused with harlequin fetus (**236**)

254 A dimple. This infant has a dimple on the posterior aspect of the shoulder. The aetiology of this finding is unknown but the mother should be persuaded that it is cosmetically attractive.

255 and 256 Stork bites. Stork bites are small capillary haemangiomata which occur classically in pairs, one over the forehead, the other over the nape of the neck. They may cause maternal concern but are of no significance and are self-limiting.

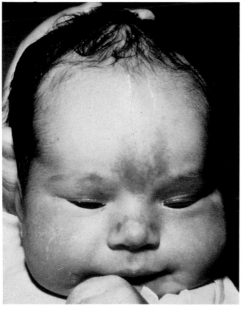

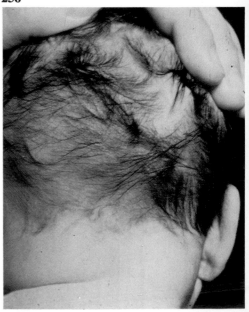

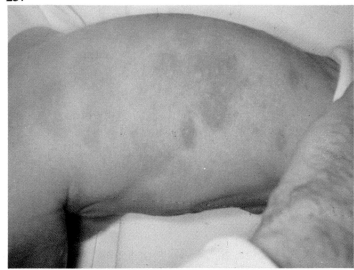

257 Toxic erythema (urticaria neonatorum). Toxic erythema is a very common rash appearing on the second or third day of life, consisting of macules with tiny white papules in the centre. It is commonly mistaken for septic spots but when the lesion is scraped and examined under the microscope only eosinophils are seen. The condition is self-limiting and harmless.

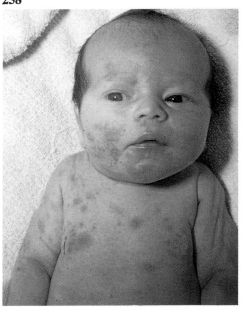

258 Urticaria neonatorum. This figure shows how the lesions of urticaria neonatorum may be extensive over the chest and face easily leading to the suspicion of skin sepsis.

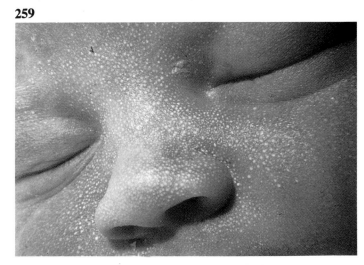

259 Milia is a common finding in new-born babies arising from obstruction of the sweat glands and involves most commonly the face, axillae and scalp. Like stork bites milia is a common cause for maternal anxiety but it too is self-limiting and does not require treatment.

260 Giant hairy naevus. A giant hairy naevus may occur anywhere in the body and is variable in size. The lesion is pigmented and is dark brown or black in colour with hairs growing from the skin over the surface which is nodular. Approximately 10% of giant hairy naevi develop into malignant melanomas.

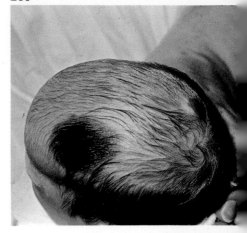
260

261 Bathing trunk naevus. This infant displays a large number of naevi of which the most dramatic is one covering the buttocks and waist posteriorly: a bathing trunk naevus. This is an extreme example of a giant hairy naevus. Treatment is difficult and may require multiple skin grafts.

261

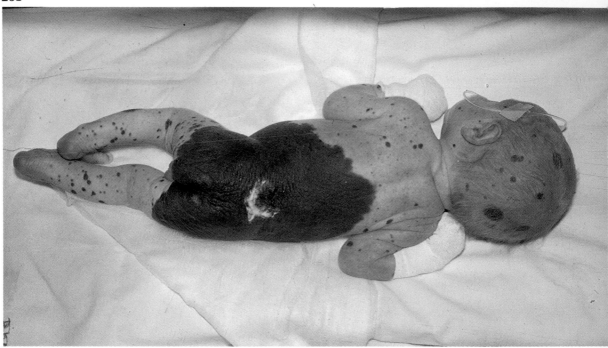

262

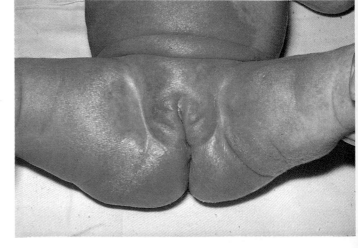

262 Ammoniacal dermatitis. When babies are left in wet nappies a dermatitis results from ammonia formed by the action of urea-splitting organisms on the skin. This commonest of nappy rashes characteristically spares the skin creases. The best treatment is exposure of the affected parts.

263 Seborrhoeic dermatitis. This rash, although superficially resembling ammoniacal dermatitis (**262**), is more extensive and has a different texture. Note that the surface of the rash is more oily and that the skin flakes on the anterior abdominal wall. Involvement of the scalp (cradle cap, **266**) is common.

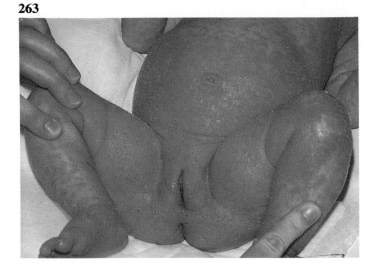

264

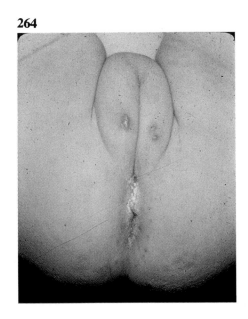

264 and 265 Monilia dermatitis. 264 illustrates isolated monilial lesions on the vulva, in the perineal area and natal cleft. This is a relatively uncommon and early presentation of a monilia nappy rash. The infant shown in **265** has a much more extensive rash which originates from the nappy area where it is confluent but which has extended to involve all of the trunk and armpits.

265

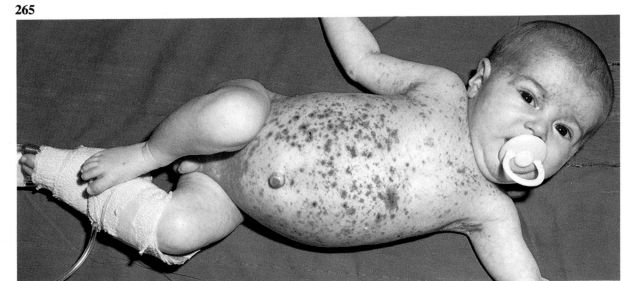

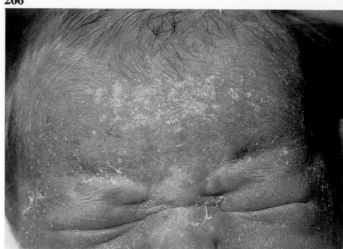

266 Cradle cap. This is the common name for seborrhoeic dermatitis involving the scalp. The greasy and flaky appearance is clearly illustrated in this figure. The mother should be reassured that the condition has no ominous significance and is self-limiting. If treatment must be given a shampoo with arachis oil helps to remove the flaky skin.

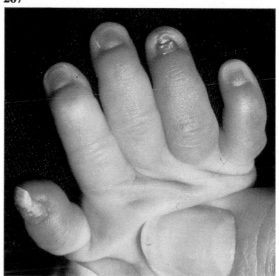

267 Monilia of the nails. This figure shows infection of the thumb and ring fingernails of the right hand due to monilia.

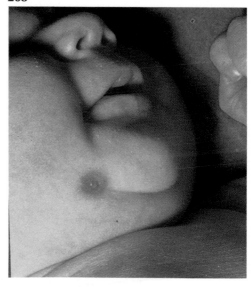

268 Pressure ulcer. This small round ulcer on the lateral aspect of the lower jaw was present at birth and was not due to prenatal infection and is believed to have been caused by pressure.

9 Genetic conditions

Genetic conditions often have characteristic phenotypes, especially in the case of chromosomal anomalies. Examples are presented to show how a constellation of abnormal physical signs, each non-specific in isolation, make a mosaic that can be diagnosed with confidence.

269

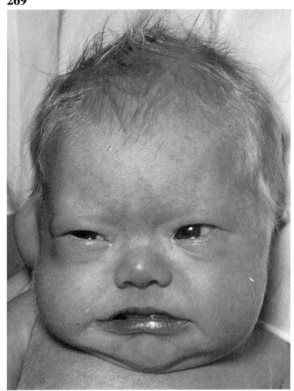

270

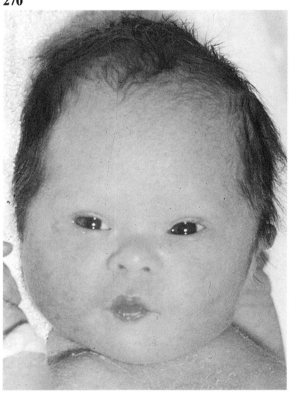

269 Down's syndrome: the face. Note the hypertelorism, broad epicanthic folds, mongoloid slant of the eyes and low set ears. The facial characteristics of Down's syndrome are sometimes less obvious in the newborn infant than in later life.

270 Down's syndrome: the face. Despite racial differences the features of Down's syndrome in this Burmese baby are similar to those seen in the Caucasian infant shown in **269**.

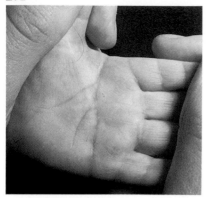

271 Down's syndrome: the hand. A single palmar crease is a classical feature of Down's syndrome and is illustrated here. A single palmar crease also occurs in other chromosomal abnormalities, but most importantly it must be remembered that it may occur as a normal variant.

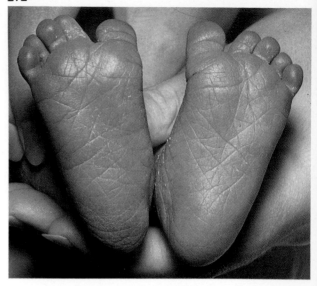

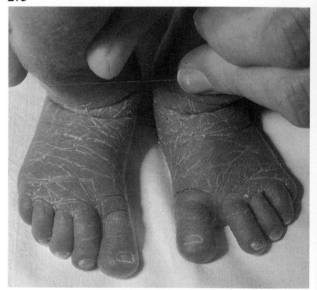

272 and 273 Down's syndrome: the foot. The plantar surface of the feet in infants with Down's syndrome show widely separated first and second toes and increased skin creases. **273** shows the dorsum of the feet of the baby illustrated in **272**.

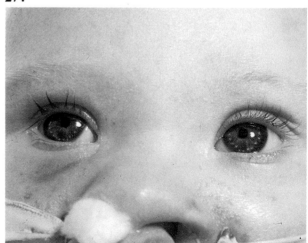

274 Down's syndrome: the eyes. Brushfield spots are another clinical characteristic of Down's syndrome. They are the tiny white spots on the iris resembling salt grains.

275 Down's syndrome: the chromosomes. This figure shows a chromosome analysis of a baby with Down's syndrome and illustrates trisomy 21 (arrow).

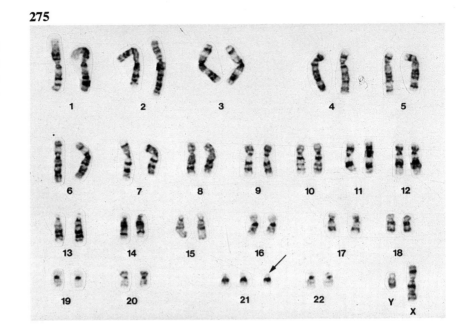

276 Mongolian spots. Mongolian spot refers to a dark blue discolouration of the lower back or buttocks and is commonly seen in infants of non-Caucasian origin. There is no relationship with Down's syndrome. Mongolian spots may be confused with bruising and this should be borne in mind when non-accidental injury is queried.

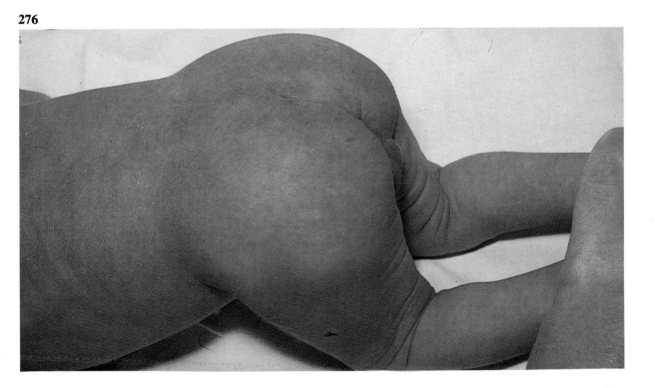

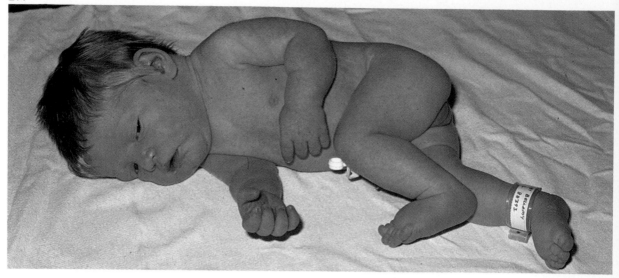

277 Turner's syndrome: the baby. Turner's syndrome is due to a genotype of 45 XO and has a variable phenotype. Patients with Turner's syndrome are female and may show no specific clinical features at birth. Sometimes, as in this case, there is lymphoedema of the feet. The infant may be light-for-dates and present with a low hairline and neck webbing.

278

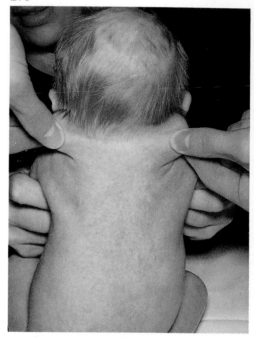

278 Turner's syndrome: the neck. This baby shows redundant skin on the postero-lateral aspect of the neck which will become a "webbed neck" as she grows older.

279 and 280 Turner's syndrome: hands and feet. These figures show lymphoedema of the hands and feet, a physical sign which should alert the clinician to consider the possible diagnosis of Turner's syndrome.

279

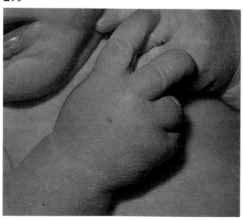

280

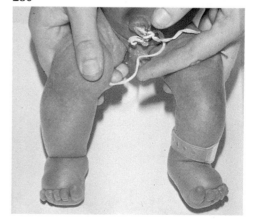

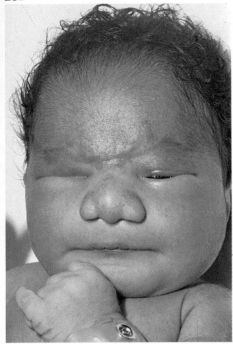

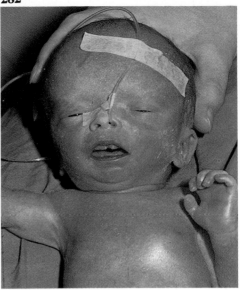

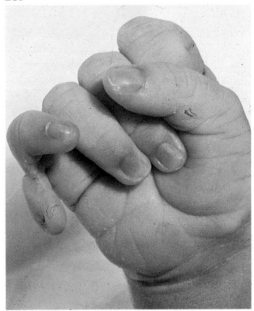

281 Patau's syndrome: the face.
Patau's syndrome is due to trisomy 13 and is the rarest of the chromosomal trisomies generally encountered. Clues from the phenotype are most obvious in the face where the broad malformed nose and microphthalmia is obvious. Colobomata and cleft palate are also common but not present in this patient.

282 Partial Patau's syndrome. Although this baby had a trisomy 13-15 on chromosomal examination, the clinical features are not classical of Patau's syndrome, hence the title.

283 Patau's syndrome: the hands. The hands in Patau's syndrome may show polydactyly and flexion deformities, a single palmar crease is the rule. Note here the extra digit and the little finger curving over the fourth finger and the fifth. These patients may also have congenital anomalies of the heart, brain and gastrointestinal tract and death before the age of 1 year is the rule.

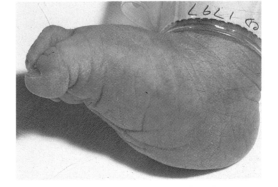

284 Patau's syndrome: the foot. A prominent heel giving rise to the term "rockerbottom foot" is often found.

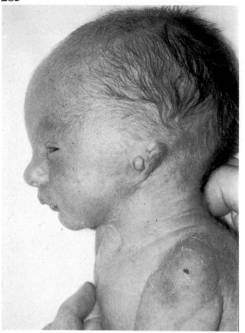

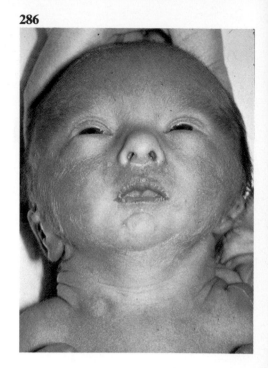

285 and 286 Edward's syndrome: the head. Edward's syndrome is due to trisomy 18. The infant is usually very small-for-dates. In this example the external ear is malformed on the left, the eyes are small and the face elfin-like. **286** is a frontal view of the same infant as illustrated in **285** demonstrating the facial characteristics.

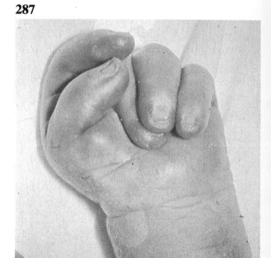

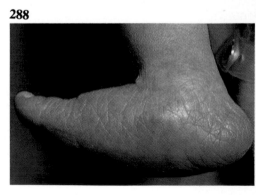

287 and 288 Edward's syndrome: the hands and feet. A characteristic of Edward's syndrome is the abnormal posture of the fingers in which the fourth and fifth fingers override the third in flexion. In **288** we see rockerbottom feet which are characteristic of Edward's syndrome as well as Patau's syndrome.

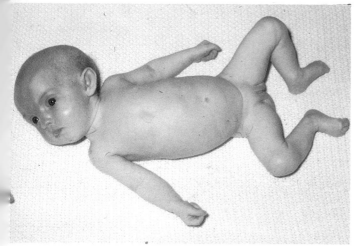

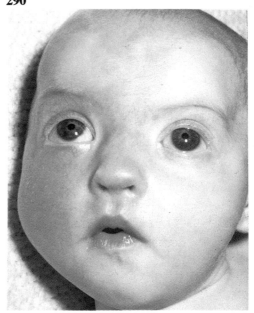

289 and 290 Wolf's syndrome refers to the phenotype associated with deletion of the short arm of chromosome 4. The distinctive characteristics of this syndrome are microcephaly, primitive ears, hypertelorism with beaking of the nose and a small downturned mouth. This infant shows in addition a coloboma of the lateral aspect of the right upper eyelid. There is poor weight gain and mental and physical retardation are manifest in later life.

292 Thanatophoric dwarf. This figure shows a stillborn infant who on superficial inspection appears to have achondroplasia. There is a group of skeletal dysplasias which are generally incompatible with life and thus known as thanatophoric dwarfism (thanatos: death).

292

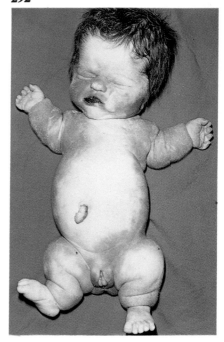

291 Achondroplasia is a dominantly inherited condition, but many cases arise by spontaneous mutation. In the neonatal period the diagnosis may be suspected in an infant who has short arms and legs with a relatively normal shaped trunk. The bulging forehead may give rise to a suspicion of hydrocephalus which occurs more commonly in patients with achondroplasia.

291

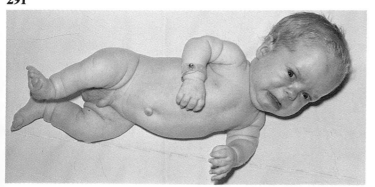

293 Rubinstein–Taybi syndrome. This rare syndrome may be diagnosed at birth by the distinctive broad thumbs and big toes. Other diagnostic features are characteristic dermatoglyphics in which the whorls on the hypothenar eminence curve away from the midline. These infants grow up to be characteristically of short stature and may be mentally handicapped.

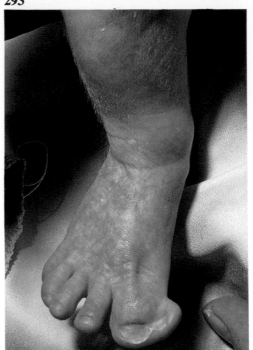

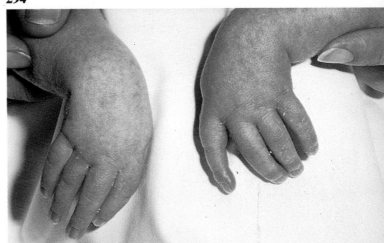

294 and 295 Arthrogryposis multiplex congenita. In arthrogryposis there is atrophy of striated muscle and thickening of joint capsules leading to rigidity and immobility of the joints. In this patient there is fixed flexion deformity with ulnar deviation of the wrists. Note also the abnormal posture of the fingers. **295** shows the ankles and feet of the patient illustrated in **294.** Note the fixed plantar flexion of the ankles. Treatment is initially by physiotherapy and subsequently orthopaedic surgery may be required.

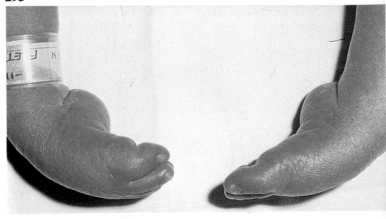

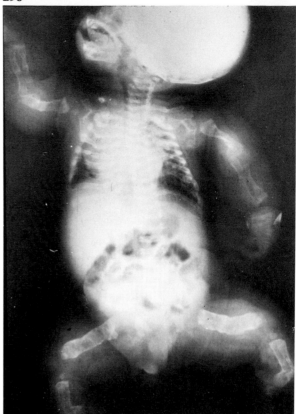

296 Osteogenesis imperfecta. This radiograph of a stillborn infant shows multiple fractures of the limb bones, a classical feature of the severest type of osteogenesis imperfecta.

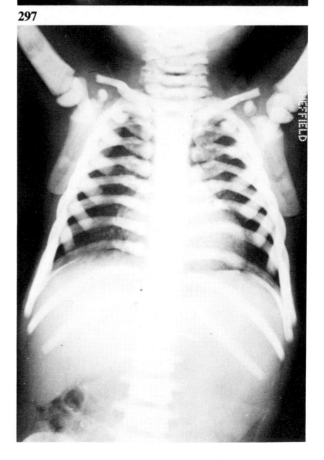

297 Osteopetrosis presenting in the newborn period is inherited as an autosomal recessive. The bones are dense, as can be seen in this radiograph, yet due to defective bone formation they are brittle. There is obliteration of the bone marrow and abnormal bone growth may lead to blindness and deafness. No treatment is available and prognosis is poor.

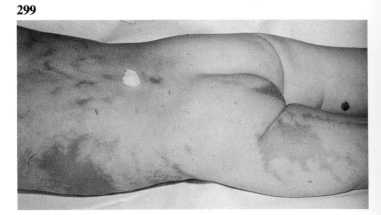

298 and 299 Incontinentia pigmenti is a multi-system disorder usually seen only in girls. The early skin lesions consist of bullae arranged in lines as shown in the figure. These occur on the trunk and limbs. The bullae may be superseded by warty lesions in the same distribution and finally after the warts disappear whorls of brown pigmentation develop in a different distribution. Many patients with incontinentia pigmenti develop abnormalities of the central nervous system such as fits or spastic paralysis. The infant shown in **299** demonstrates the pigmented whorls characteristic of incontinentia pigmenti. In this case the whorls appeared without the prior development of bullae or warts.

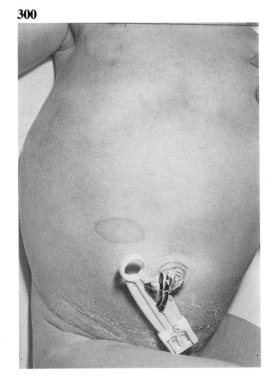

300 Neurofibromatosis is an autosomal dominant condition involving principally the skin and central nervous system. The diagnosis may be suspected in the newborn by the presence of ''cafe au lait'' spots seen here on the right side of the abdomen.

301 and 302 Cystic fibrosis is a recessively inherited disorder occurring in approximately 1 in 2500 Caucasian births. The disease may be manifest before birth resulting in meconium ileus. The meconium is abnormally sticky resulting in intestinal blockage and peritonitis. The meconium may calcify. In **301** there is abdominal distension without fluid levels. A rarer presentation of cystic fibrosis in the newborn is pneumonia, seen in the chest radiograph illustrated in **302**.

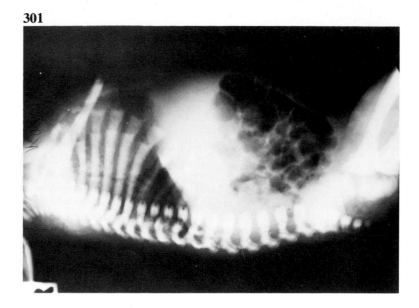

301

302

303 Meconium plug. The sticky meconium in cystic fibrosis may be passed as a long plug of material as seen in this specimen.

303

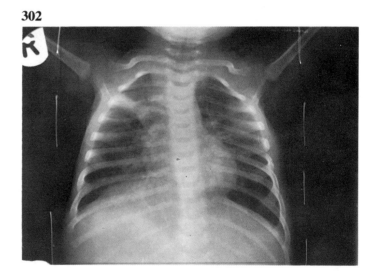

10 Conditions acquired prenatally

Much of the pathology seen after birth has had its origin before birth and many of the examples shown in other chapters could also be placed under the title of "conditions acquired prenatally". This chapter concentrates on prenatal infections that maim but do not kill the fetus, on the effects of prenatal exposure to drugs and on the consequence of transfer of antibodies from mother to fetus. We begin with prenatal infection.

304

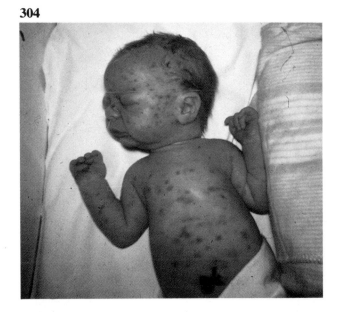

305

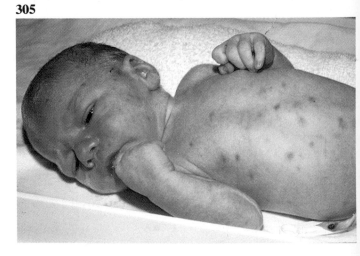

304 and 305 Congenital rubella: purpura. Maternal rubella in the first trimester may be associated with teratogenic malformations in the fetus. The sequelae depend on when maternal infection occurred and include microcephaly, deafness, blindness and congenital cardiac malformation. This infant presented as a small-for-dates baby with a purpuric rash due to thrombocytopaenia. Such a clinical presentation should arouse the paediatrician's suspicion of prenatal viral infection and appropriate steps should be taken to protect the other patients and staff since the infant is likely to remain a source of contagion. **305** is a further illustration of the purpuric rash due to congenital rubella. The differential diagnosis includes other prenatally acquired infections, septicaemia and disseminated intravascular coagulation.

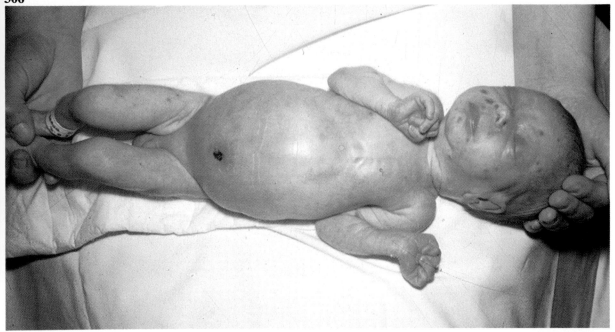

306 Congenital rubella: hepatospleno-megaly. Another clinical clue to prenatal infection is unexplained hepatospleno-megaly. This baby has a distended abdomen due to hepatosplenomegaly and ascites (see also **198**).

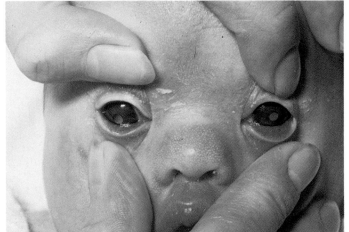

307 Congenital rubella: cataracts. This figure shows the cataracts that may occur in infants with congenital rubella.

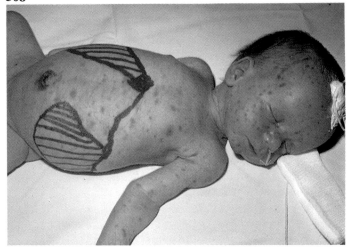

308 Congenital cytomegalovirus infection. This infant shows huge splenomegaly, hepatomegaly and a purpuric rash and illustrates the diagnostic problem facing the clinician since there is no clinical way of being sure which prenatal virus caused the physical sign.

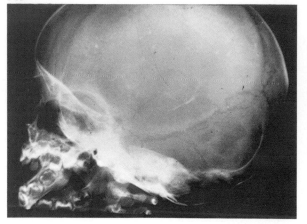

309 Congenital toxoplasmosis: skull radiograph. Prenatal infection with the protozoan *Toxoplasma gondii* may resemble prenatal viral infection but this radiograph illustrates the importance of performing a skull X-ray as part of the initial investigations of such infants since there is diffuse cerebral calcification characteristic of toxoplasmosis. Cerebral calcification may be associated subsequently with hydrocephaly or microcephaly.

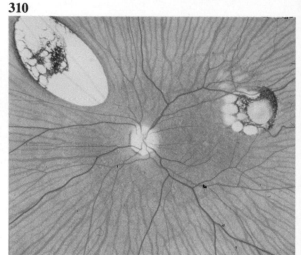

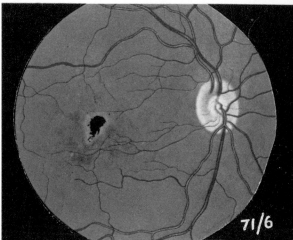

310 and 311 Congenital toxoplasmosis: optic fundus. Examination of the optic fundus may reveal changes in the neonatal period as shown in this painting which illustrates a patch of chorioretinitis at the macula. Later in childhood the chorioretinitis proceeds to produce characteristic scars as seen in **311**.

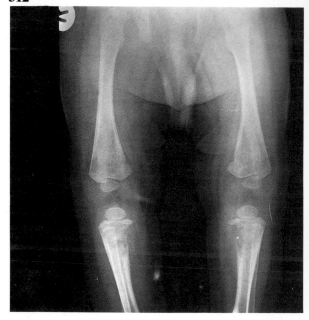

312 Congenital syphilis. Congenital syphilis is now rare but presents clinically with a florid nasal discharge followed by a copper coloured rash particularly in the muco-cutaneous areas. This radiograph shows the classical osteochrondritis and periosteal thickening of the long bones in a newborn infant with congenital syphilis.

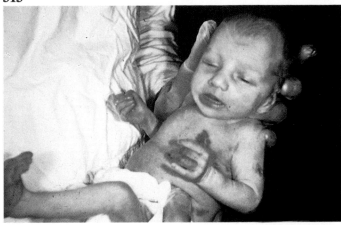

313

313 Congenital herpes. Herpes simplex may be acquired as the fetus passes through the birth canal. The disease becomes widespread due to lack of immune defence and involves the liver, adrenals and lungs leading to jaundice, hepatomegaly and dyspnoea. The brain may be involved. There is a characteristic vesicular skin rash seen in this figure. Prognosis is poor but the development of effective anti-herpetic therapy may improve the outlook.

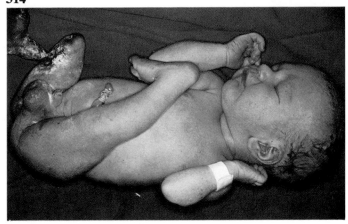

314

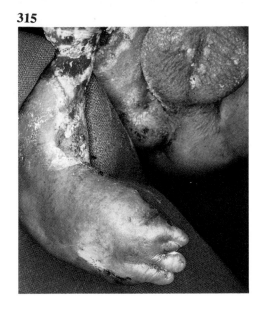

315

314 and 315 Congenital varicella. Maternal infection with varicella during the first trimester has been reported to cause fetal malformations including reduction deformities of a limb and scars along the length of the affected limbs. In addition the infant may be small-for-dates and demonstrate features of central nervous system involvement including encephalitis and chorioretinitis. This syndrome is not to be confused with congenital herpes infection (see **313**) which is acquired by direct contact with the virus in the birth canal.

No pregnant woman should be given drug therapy without balancing the fetal risk against maternal benefit as the examples overleaf illustrate.

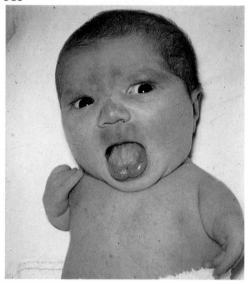

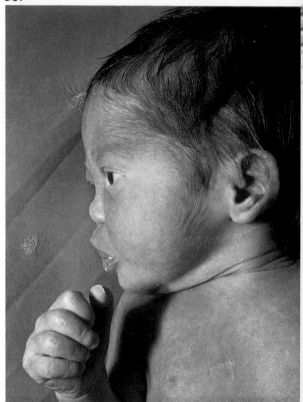

316 Thalidomide baby. Thalidomide is the classical example of teratogenesis resulting from drug ingestion. This particular drug was taken as a mild sedative until it was discovered that phocomelia and amelia of the fetus resulted. This figure shows a baby with grossly foreshortened arms, an example of phocomelia.

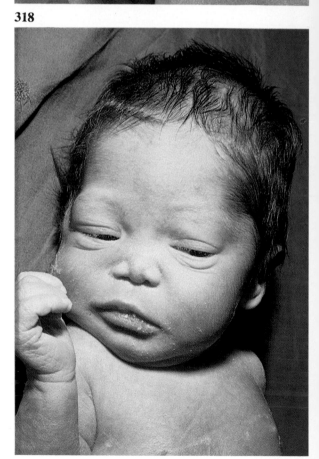

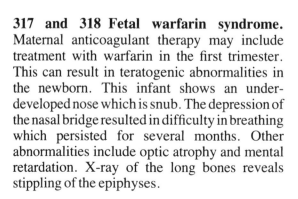

317 and 318 Fetal warfarin syndrome. Maternal anticoagulant therapy may include treatment with warfarin in the first trimester. This can result in teratogenic abnormalities in the newborn. This infant shows an underdeveloped nose which is snub. The depression of the nasal bridge resulted in difficulty in breathing which persisted for several months. Other abnormalities include optic atrophy and mental retardation. X-ray of the long bones reveals stippling of the epiphyses.

319

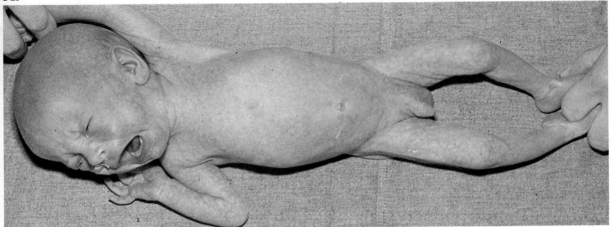

319 Maternal diazoxide therapy. Diazoxide may be used as a hypotensive during pregnancy. The drug crosses the placenta and patients treated in this way gave rise to concern because of possible hypotensive or diabetogenic effects on the fetus. The only clinical sequel observed was total alopecia.

320

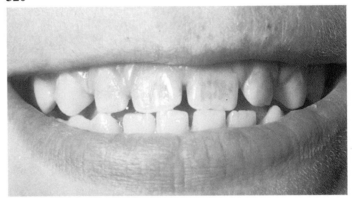

320 Tetracycline stained teeth. If tetracyclines are given during pregnancy or in the neonatal period staining of the permanent teeth results leading to an unsightly brown discolouration as seen in this figure and abnormal enamel formation.

321

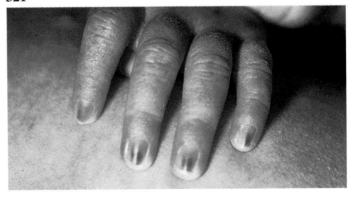

321 Tetracycline nail staining. In the same way tetracycline may result in staining of the nails of the newborn. Unlike the teeth, staining of the nails is happily self-limiting.

322

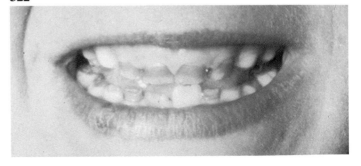

322 Teeth staining. Staining of the teeth is not always due to tetracycline and can also arise due to neonatal hyperbilirubinaemia.

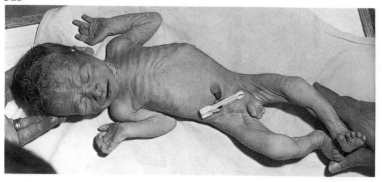

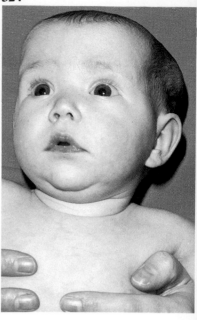

323 Transient diabetes mellitus. Transient diabetes mellitus is a rare neonatal problem which should be suspected when a grossly small-for-dates baby fails to gain weight despite having a voracious appetite. Careful review will show that the infant is polyuric and glycosuric. Treatment with insulin is necessary. The condition remits spontaneously after a period of weeks to months. The aetiology remains a mystery.

324 Neonatal thyrotoxicosis. Newborn infants may have a temporary thyrotoxicosis due to transplacental passage of long-acting thyroid stimulator (LATS). This baby is unnaturally alert and shows a slight degree of exophthalmos. Palpation of the neck revealed a small, diffuse goitre. Thyrotoxicosis in the newborn may be lethal due to cardiac decompensation and treatment with antithyroid drugs and betablockers is usually necessary.

There is a small group of conditions which arise from the transfer of antibodies from mother to fetus. These include transient thrombocytopenic purpura, which looks like any other purpura (see **346**) until a careful history is taken, transient myaesthenia gravis, which is not photogenic and neonatal thyrotoxicosis.

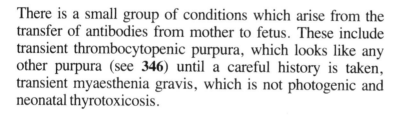

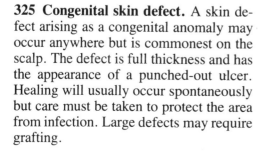

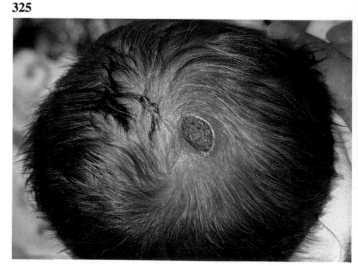

325 Congenital skin defect. A skin defect arising as a congenital anomaly may occur anywhere but is commonest on the scalp. The defect is full thickness and has the appearance of a punched-out ulcer. Healing will usually occur spontaneously but care must be taken to protect the area from infection. Large defects may require grafting.

11 Conditions acquired postnatally

326

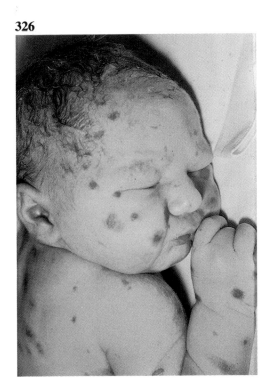

327

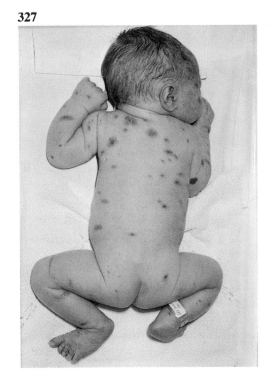

326 and 327 Urticaria pigmentosa is caused by mast cell infiltration of the skin. The rash may be an isolated lesion or diffuse as shown in these figures. Histamine release results in itching, flushing, tachycardia and irritability. Occasionally mast cell infiltration may affect the liver, spleen and bone marrow in which case the outlook is poor. The skin lesions usually resolve spontaneously.

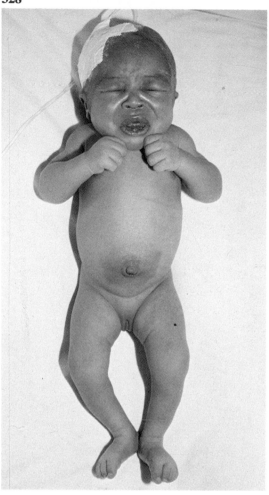

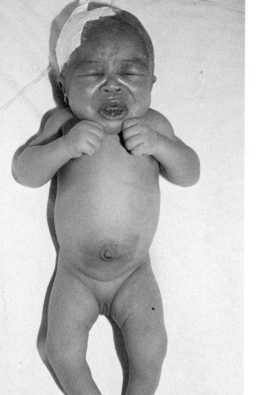

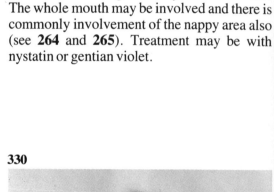

329 Oral thrush. Infection of the oropharynx with candida is common in the first weeks of life. Oral thrush is distinguished from milk curds by being difficult to detach from the mucosa and leaving a raw erythematous base. The whole mouth may be involved and there is commonly involvement of the nappy area also (see **264** and **265**). Treatment may be with nystatin or gentian violet.

328 Neonatal tetanus. This figure is practically diagnostic of neonatal tetanus. Tetanus has resulted from unclean handling of the umbilical cord; note the inflammation around the umbilicus. The classical features of tetanus; trismus, risus sardonicus and muscle spasms of the arms and legs are also apparent.

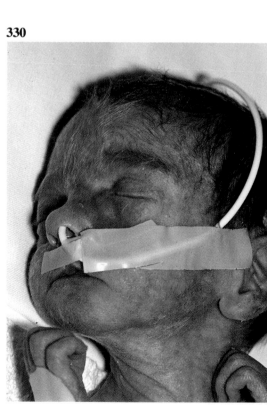

330 Dacrocystitis. This pre-term infant has an inflamed swelling between the nose and inner corner of the left eye due to infection of the lacrimal duct (see also **76**).

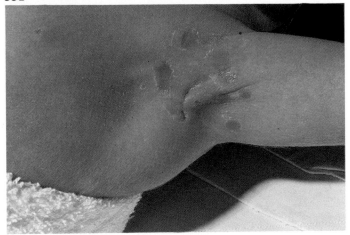

331

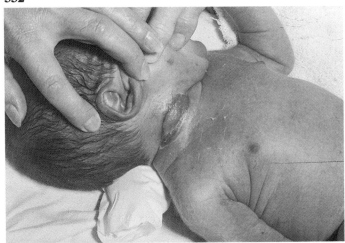

332

331 and 332 Neonatal impetigo.
Neonatal impetigo is usually due to staphylococcal infection and may run in epidemics in newborn nurseries. The organism seeks warm, moist areas such as the axillae as shown in **332**, or the folds of the neck or groins. The lesions are superficial blisters or ulcers. In **332** the impetigo is affecting the skin creases of the neck.

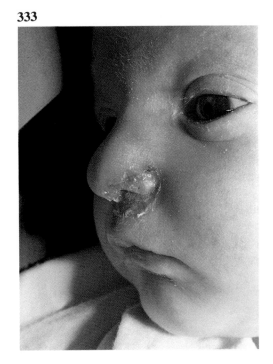

333

333 Neonatal impetigo. *Staphylococcus aureus* is commonly found in nasal swabs and is usually a commensal organism. In this infant the organism was virulent and caused extensive local ulceration and crusting. The treatment of neonatal impetigo should be both local and systemic because of the risk of septicaemic spread. Babies with impetigo should be isolated.

334

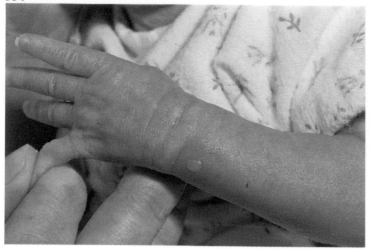

335

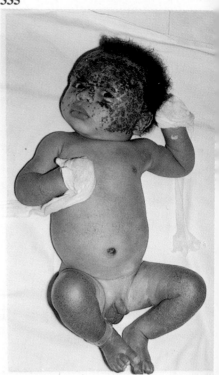

334 Septic spot. This infant had a septic, fluid-filled spot on the dorsal aspect of the wrist. Found as an isolated lesion this should alert the clinician to the possibility of prenatal or postnatal acquired infection.

336

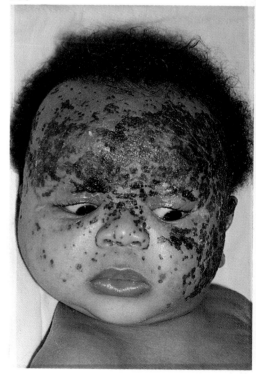

335 and 336 Herpes simplex, postnatally acquired. This baby was treated with topical steroids for a postnatal skin lesion which turned out to be herpes simplex. The herpes became exfoliative and involved widespread areas of the skin of the face as seen in the figure.

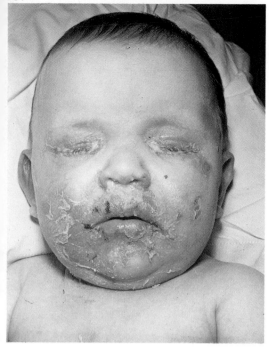

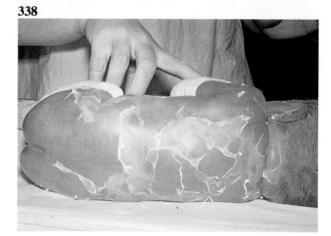

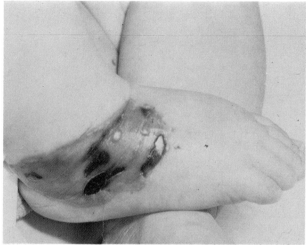

337 and 338 Toxic epidermal necrolysis.
Toxic epidermal necrolysis is the severest form of superficial staphylococcal infection in the newborn. It may start suddenly and progress rapidly. The face is affected first, showing initially erythema, crusting and bullae. Progression may become rapidly generalized. In **338** there is widespread infection of the back with exfoliation of the skin which peels on touch.

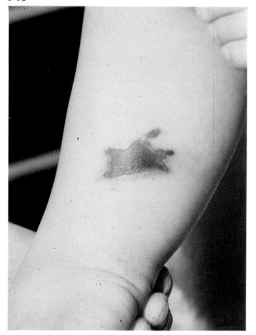

339 and 340 Ecchymosis. This may occur with purpura with any form of disseminated intravascular coagulation. The commonest cause in the newborn is septicaemia; this baby had a Haemophilus septicaemia and meningitis.

341

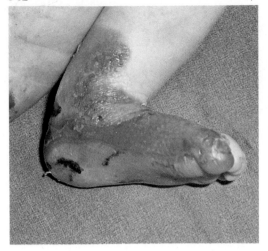

342

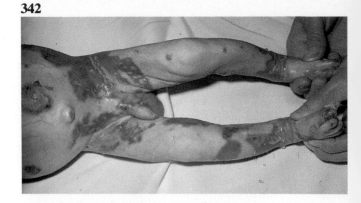

343

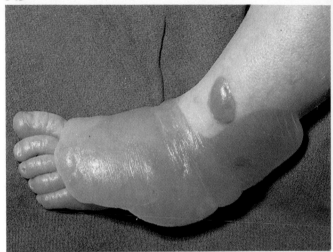

341, 342 and 343 Epidermolysis bullosa.
Epidermolysis bullosa is a generic term applied to a group of conditions all inherited autosomally in which the skin blisters or sheds at the slightest trauma. The foot is one of the most commonly affected sites because babies kick their feet. In the infant illustrated in **342** there is widespread involvement. In some cases healing is complete, but in others scarring may result. **343** illustrates an early stage in the illness in which there is blister formation on the lateral aspect of the foot of recent onset. The blister will burst with the slightest trauma.

344

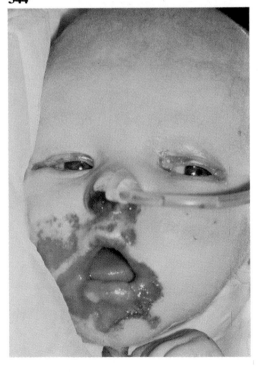

344 Essential fatty acid deficiency. Total parenteral nutrition may result in essential fatty acid deficiency which causes erythematous scaling rashes similar to those seen in epidermolysis bullosa. The two should be considered an alternative differential diagnoses.

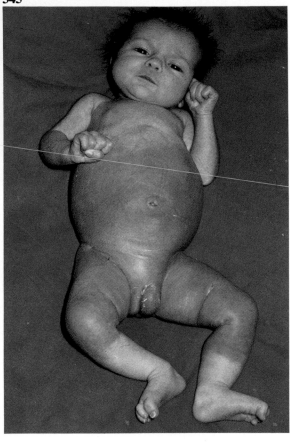

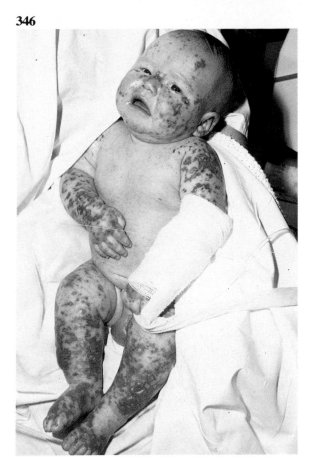

345 Erysipelas. The term erysipelas is used to denote a rapidly spreading cellulitis caused by beta haemolytic streptococcal infection. The lesion classically has a distinct edge which may be raised. The involved skin is erythematous and thickened. Response to penicillin therapy is usually excellent although occasionally the disease may spread so rapidly that it is fatal.

347

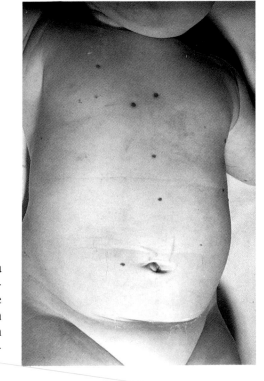

346 and 347 Purpura. The baby illustrated in **346** shows a widespread purpuric rash involving the limbs and face particularly. This was due to meningococcal infection but may be associated with septicaemia from any organism. The infant in **347** has many fewer purpuric spots but is also suffering from septicaemia. Purpura is an ominous clinical sign in any newborn infant and should be analysed speedily and carefully.

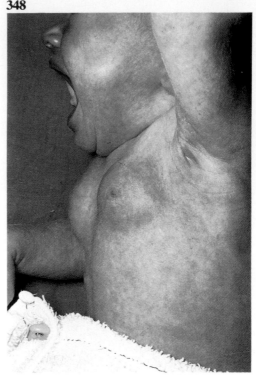

348 Neonatal mastitis. Breast enlargement is common in babies and results from transplacental transfer to the fetus of maternal oestrogens. Milk (witch's milk) may be secreted. The swelling subsides spontaneously in a few weeks. The mother and other potentially meddlesome relatives must not try to relieve the swelling by expressing the milk since infection will almost certainly follow (see **349**).

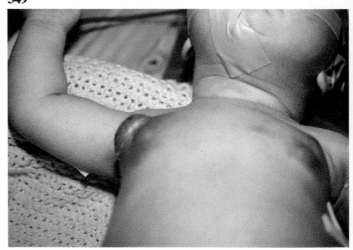

349 Neonatal breast abscess. Superinfection of neonatal mastitis may result in breast abscess formation as seen in this figure. Treatment is by surgical drainage.

12 Trauma

350 and 351 Skull fracture. Fracture of the skull may result from birth trauma. The neonatal skull is thin and pliable and thus should be handled with care. This infant shows extensive facial bruising and a depressed fracture over the left frontal area. Opinion is divided as to whether treatment should be passive or involve surgical lifting of the fracture. The radiograph shown in **351** illustrates a large parieto-occipital fracture with extensive soft tissue swelling.

350

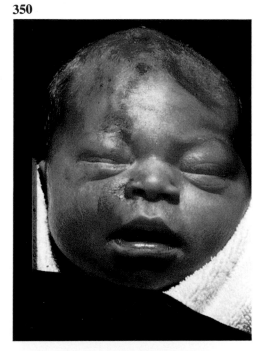

351

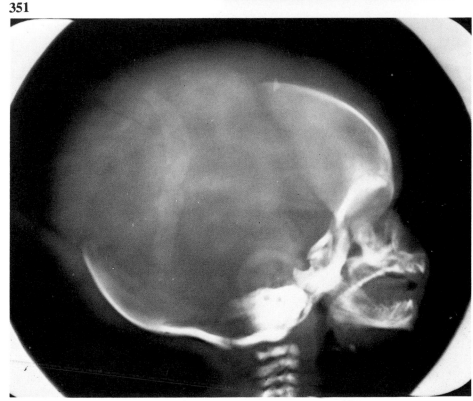

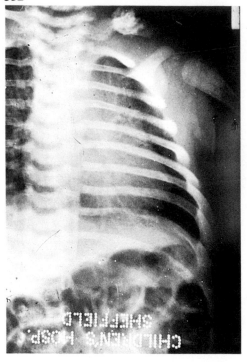

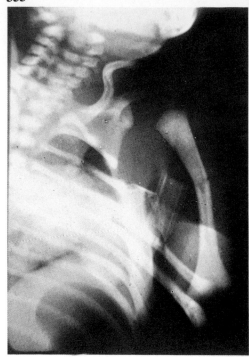

352 Fracture of clavicle. The clavicle is the commonest bone fractured during delivery. Trauma may result from shoulder dystocia. The baby is often asymptomatic and the first clinical sign may be a lump over the clavicle resulting from callus formation.

353 Fracture of humerus. This too may arise as a result of shoulder dystocia and may be associated with lesions of the brachial plexus due to traction on the shoulder girdle. The upper arm is swollen, painful and immobile.

354

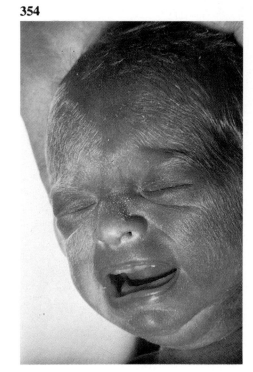

354 Facial bruising. Bruising of the face may occur and particularly affects pre-term infants who are more prone to abnormal presentation; face or breech. This baby of 31 weeks gestation was a face presentation.

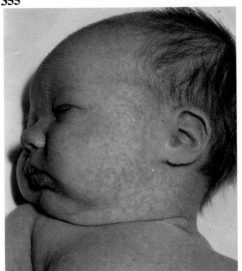

355

355 Facial petechiae. Petechiae are commonly seen on the face in babies who are born with the umbilical cord round the neck or in whom there is abnormal delay following delivery of the head and neck before the trunk and shoulders are delivered. Facial petechiae, along with subconjunctival haemorrhage, do not have the same ominous significance as petechiae on the trunk and limbs and fade in the first few days of life. In this figure the baby has been photographed at the age of 2 days when the petechiae already resemble freckles.

356

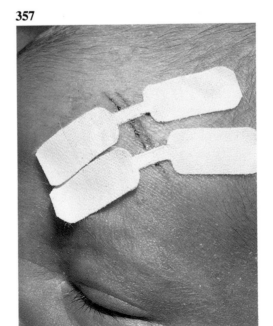

356 Bruising of tongue. This rare complication may arise from traumatic resuscitation. If severe the baby may be unwilling to feed and experience difficulty in breathing due to swelling blocking the oro-pharynx. Naso-gastric feeding may be necessary.

357

357 Scalp laceration. Laceration of any part of the baby may occur if the infant is born by enthusiastic caesarean section. On this occasion the cut was superficial and on the forehead.

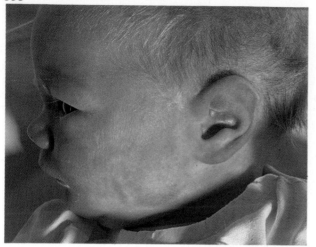

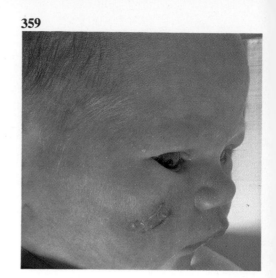

358 and 359 Forceps marks. Forceps marks on the cheek are common and are a reassuring sign that the forceps blades were applied correctly. Rarely a temporary facial nerve palsy may be associated. Occasionally the forceps may actually traumatize the skin leading to ulceration. The baby shown in **359** also had a facial palsy.

360 Cephalhaematoma: clinical. Cephalhaematoma is a sub-periosteal haemorrhage caused by birth trauma. It should be distinguished from caput succudaneum because it is confined by the suture lines of the bone over which it lies. Cephalhaematoma causes parental concern but reassurance should be given, even though a rim of new bone may form where the periosteum had been stripped away from the skull. This too will resolve as the child grows up.

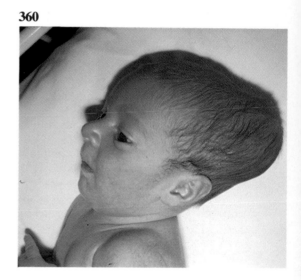

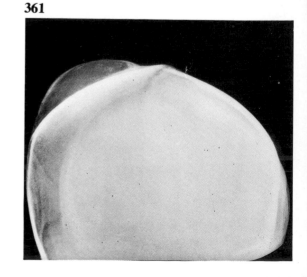

361 Cephalhaematoma: radiograph. This radiograph shows a cephalhaematoma in profile and illustrates the periosteal new bone that may form around the perimeter of the lesion.

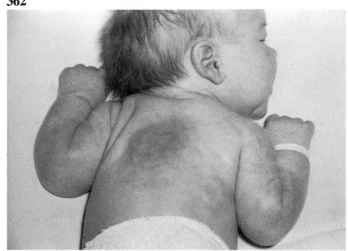

362

362 Subcutaneous fat necrosis is rarely seen now but has previously been associated with cold injuries in the newborn or shock. In this infant there was a purple indurated area over the small of the back which was thought to be septic. On incision necrotic fatty tissue was aspirated. If managed conservatively, spontaneous healing usually occurs.

363

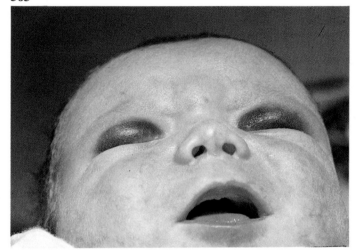

363 Periorbital bruising. This infant has two black eyes. Orbital bruising may result from fractures of the anterior fossa and also in subdural haematoma. In each case blood tracks down to the periorbital area from the site of the inital bleed.

364

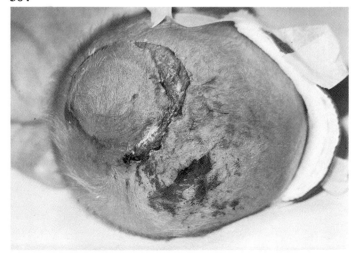

364 Vacuum extractor chignon. The word chignon refers to the localized area of scalp oedema caused by the suction of the cup applied during a ventouse extraction. Most cases resolve spontaneously but if associated with perinatal asphyxia there may be necrosis of the chignon leading to ulceration of the scalp.

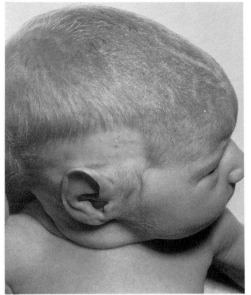

365 Subaponeurotic haemorrhage is a rare complication of ventouse extraction in which there is bleeding into the subaponeurotic space. The loss of blood may be large leading to hypovolaemia and shock.

366 Bruised buttocks should not be confused with Mongolian blue spots (see **276**) but are a complication of breech delivery. The loss of blood into the buttocks may be enough to cause hypovolaemia and when seen in pre-term infants a significant jaundice often results. Male infants with bruised buttocks may also have testicular trauma.

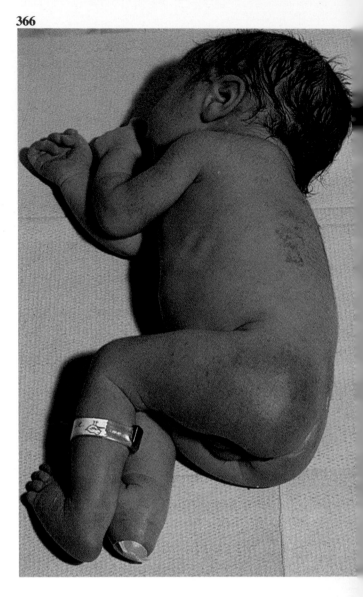

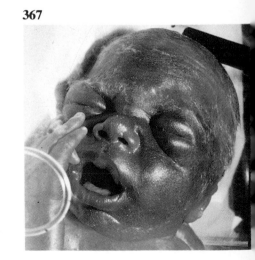

367 Bruised face. This figure shows the gross facial bruising that may follow a difficult delivery.

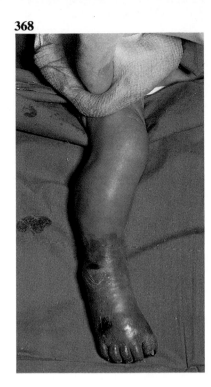

368 Gangrenous leg. This infant has developed gangrene of the right foot and leg due to a femoral artery embolus following umbilical artery catheterization. Through knee amputation resulted.

369 Cardiac catheter. This infant has the tip of an umbilical venous catheter in the right side of the heart (arrow). This unfortunate complication arose due to transection of the umbilical cord with an umbilical catheter *in situ* followed by unsuccessful exploration which resulted in the catheter tip being pushed into the portal vein whence it disappeared via the ductus venosus to lodge in the heart.

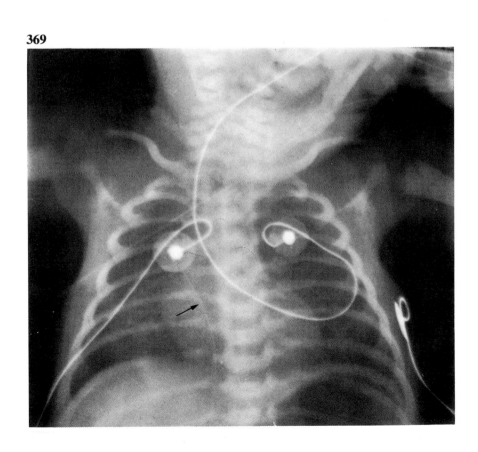

Further reading

Textbooks

Avery, G.B. (1981) *Neonatology and Pathophysiology of the Newborn* J.B. Lippincott (Philadelphia).

Schaffer, A.J. and Avery, M.E. (1977) *Diseases of the Newborn.* W.B. Saunders (Philadephia).

Short monographs

Babson, S.G., Pernoll, M.L. and Benda, G.I. (1980) *Diagnosis and Management of the Fetus and Neonate at Risk.* C.V. Mosby (St Louis).

Brown, R.J.K. and Valman, H.B. (1979) *Practical Neonatal Paediatrics.* Blackwell Scientific Publications (Oxford).

Roberton, N.R.C. (1981) *Manual of Neonatal Intensive Care.* Edward Arnold (London).

References to specific slides

314: Savage, M.O., Moosa, A. and Gordon, R.R. (1973) Maternal varicella infection as a cause of fetal malformations. *Lancet* **i**, 352–354.

317: Milner, R.D.G. and Chouksey, S.K. (1972) Effect of fetal exposure to diazoxide in man. *Archives of Diseases in Childhood* **47**, 537–544.

Index

135